ADVANCE PRAISE FOR
THE WAY OF THE ICEMAN

"After teaching specialized breathing techniques to SEALs for years, helping them focus, stay warm in the cold ocean and get centered in combat, I can attest to the authenticity and power of Wim Hof's methods. Wim Hof is providing a great service with his new book *The Way of The Iceman* by bringing breath training and simple, powerful health practices into mainstream consciousness."

—**MARK DIVINE**, US Navy SEAL (ret), Founder
SEALFIT, Best-selling author of *Unbeatable Mind* and
Way of the SEAL

"Homo sapiens is a species that is uniquely and tragically ill-adapted to our environment. Maladies ranging from heart disease to diabetes to autoimmune disorders are generated by the mismatch between the natural world we evolved to live in and the artificial realms in which we find ourselves today. Wim Hof's teachings show us how to recalibrate our bodies in a way that recognizes the extremes of our natural environment as teachers to be celebrated and consulted, rather than enemies to be insulated against. Wim's deepest insights resonate with our hunter-gatherer ancestors, who understood the wisdom of adapting to the natural world rather than trying to dominate and control it."

—**CHRISTOPHER RYAN**, PhD., New York Times best-selling author of *Sex at Dawn*

"I am continuously searching for ways to expand my mind, body and spirit—Wim Hof and *The Way of The Iceman* have done just that! He shows us that human potential is limitless and we are ALL capable of anything we set our minds to."

—LEWIS HOWES, New York Times best-selling author of *The School of Greatness*

"What fascinates me most about Wim Hof's method is the potential application for athletes...the science in this book shows that we can all amplify our recovery, maximize our pain tolerance, massively jack up energy levels and even learn to control inflammation...and it can be done *without* resorting to toxic drugs. In fact, the system outlined in this manual might just be the key to producing a generation of enhanced *but drug-free* athletes."

—PAUL "COACH" WADE, author of *Convict Conditioning*

"We live in a chaotic modern world with daily assaults on our health from frenetic schedules, poor sleep, high stress, chronic disease, and infectious illness. Our brain and nervous system have been highjacked by this toxic environment, always on high alert with real consequences to our physical and mental health.

With *The Way of The Iceman*, Wim Hof has given a profound gift to public health. The science is solid and the results actual and measureable. As you follow his remarkable life story it is readily apparent that this man is no charlatan or snake oil salesman.

Through years of commitment and self-experimentation, Wim has empirically figured out how to exert significant control over the autonomic nervous system, a feat once thought impossible. His method has held up to scrutiny under the dispassionate lens of science, expanding our knowledge of what is possible with dedicated training in what is now known as the Wim Hof Method.

Deceptively simple, and incredibly powerful, *The Way of the Iceman* gives you not only the scientific framework, but actionable steps you can implement to take back control over your high-jacked brain, increase resilience from illness, and start healing yourself from the inside out. The Wim Hof Method has become a cornerstone in my personal daily wellness plan, and as a public health physician, I cannot recommend it highly enough."

—**DR. CHRIS HARDY**, D.O. MPH, CSCS, Public Health Physician, Integrative Medicine Specialis, author of *Strong Medicine*

"*The Way of The Iceman* is one of only two books in my life that I have read cover to cover the first time I put my hands on it.

What won me over was the simplicity of the explanations of diabetes, inflammation and the family of modern ills. Moreover, the discussion on diet, just a brief mention of 'Fast-Five,' is the first time I actually understood not only how inflammation is such an issue, but a means to deal with it.

This book is the missing link for most of us: the discussion of breathing is so simple, yet so doable; coaches and athletes will understand a newer and simpler means of recovery.

Nothing in the book is over the top and we are talking about a guy who swims under ice. The method is so simple, yet so elegant. It's marvelous and I think you will apply the techniques immediately."

—**DANIEL JOHN**, author of *Never Let Go*

"Wim Hof has learned to control his physiology in a way rarely seen in human history. This book takes his extraordinary techniques and simplifies them so you can optimize your health and wellness. I recommend you learn the unique methods Wim has mastered in order to add vitality to your body and life."

—**CHAD WATERBURY**, neurophysiologist, author of *The Muscle Revolution*

"I found The Way of The Iceman absolutely fascinating! Many of us are familiar with the numerous benefits of cold training, such as increased energy levels, better circulation and improved mood, but nothing on the subject has ever been presented of this magnitude before! The legend himself, Wim Hof, along with Koen De Jong, share not only a detailed account of Mr. Hof's lifetime achievements (such as running a marathon in the Arctic… in just a pair of shorts!), but also practical, actionable methods that anyone can employ.

This book has everything from progressive cold submersion methods to breathing techniques. It delves into meditation and spirituality, but also presents the hard science to back it up.

Any fan of physical culture or anybody curious about how far the human limits can be pushed needs to add this to their library."

—**DANNY KAVADLO**, author of *Strength Rules*

"Wim Hof's techniques healed my gut where nothing else would. And I tried everything. *The Way of The Iceman* should be required reading. The world is just beginning to realize the extraordinary gift we have in Wim Hof."

—**MARK JOYNER**, founder of Simpleology

"As someone who enjoys bare-chested, outdoor winter calisthenics workouts, Wim Hof's extreme cold weather feats immediately appealed to me.

The Wim Hof Method is so simple that anyone can get started right away. And the results are so palpable that once you start, you'll almost certainly want to keep going."

—**AL KAVADLO**, author of *Street Workout* and *Pushing The Limits!*

"Wim Hof first came across my radar a few years ago when I heard of a crazy Dutchman defying the laws of thermodynamics. How could a man submerge himself in freezing water for prolonged periods of time without hypothermia? How was it possible for his body temperature to stay the same during the process?

This book is an enlightening look into the nervous system, and the amazing power of the mind. Don't mistake this for simple 'cold therapy' although that is a piece of the puzzle.

This book will give you a front row seat to an education on the nervous system, and how one man and his disciples have learned to control it in a way that we previously thought was impossible.

I found *The Way of The Iceman* fascinating."

—**MAX SHANK**, founder of Ultimate Athleticism and author of *Master The Kettlebell*

When I read *The Way of The Iceman* I was struck with awe and hope! Wim has brought scientific evidence to what I personally believe and have been teaching my students for years about breathing, bioenergetics and our connection to the spirit world. By demystifying the religious Wim is helping to support a Truth in the New World; mainly that spirituality without science descends into superstition, and science without spirituality degrades humanity into the meaninglessness of materialism."

—**ELLIOTT HULSE**

THE WAY OF
THE ICEMAN

© 2016, Dragon Door Publications, Inc
A Dragon Door Publications, Inc. production
All rights under International and Pan-American Copyright conventions.
Published in the United States by: Dragon Door Publications, Inc.
5 East County Rd B, #3 | Little Canada, MN 55117
Tel: (651) 487-2180 | Fax: (651) 487-3954
Credit card orders: 1-800-899-5111 | Email: support@dragondoor.com
Website: www.dragondoor.com

ISBN-10: 1-9428- 1209-4 | ISBN-13: 978-1- 9428-1209- 8
This edition first published in February, 2017
Printed in China

The Dutch original was published in 2016 by Uitgeverij Lucht BV, Nederhorst Den Berg,
under the title Koud Kunstje. © Wim Hof and Koen de Jong.
All rights reserved.

Translation from Dutch to English by Andy Brown

Book and cover design by Derek Brigham | www.dbrigham.com | bigd@dbrigham.com

Photograph on Page 36 by Peter Schagen
Photograph of Koen de Jong by Michel Porro
All other photographs by Enahm Hof

DISCLAIMER: The authors and publisher of this material are not responsible in any manner whatsoever for
any injury that may occur through following the instructions contained in this material. The activities, physical
and otherwise, described herein for informational purposes only, may be too strenuous or dangerous for
some people and the reader(s) should consult a physician before engaging in them. The content of this book
is for informational and educational purposes only and should not be considered medical advice, diagnosis, or
treatment. Readers should not disregard, or delay in obtaining, medical advice for any medical condition they
may have, and should seek the assistance of their health care professionals for any such conditions because of
information contained within this publication.

CONTENTS

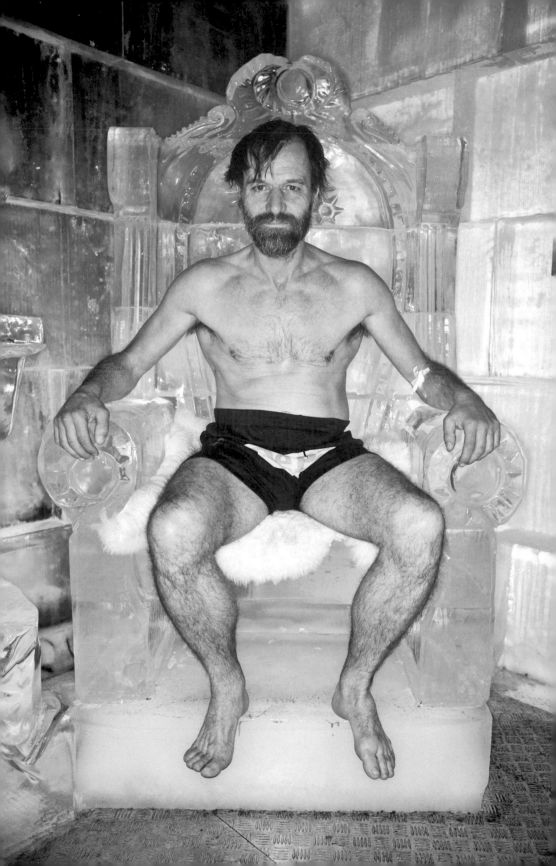

FOREWORD TO THE ENGLISH EDITION

BY JESSE ITZLER

Do you remember in the summer of 2014, when the ALS Ice Bucket Challenge went viral on social media? Yeah, so do I. There were all kinds of videos posted of friends, family, celebrities and random strangers. They'd take a bucket of ice and water, place it over their heads and then turn it upside down. The results were almost always the same—when the freezing water hit the skin of those being challenged they would let out a high-pitch squealing noise and then run off into the woods somewhere. Admittedly, I did the same thing.

Over 17 million people participated in the challenge, but as far as I know nobody "nominated" Wim Hof. Why would they? An ice bucket of water dumped on Wim is a stroll in the park. I mean...a dump truck of ice poured on Wim wouldn't be challenging. In fact, it's welcoming! It's his happy place. Wim has taken what we consider "hard" or uncomfortable and flipped that bucket upside down. He has made a living getting comfortable being uncomfortable—and it's not because he was originally wired differently from the rest of us. It's because he invested the time to re-wire himself differently.

Perhaps you've seen him on television swimming in ice-cold waters, going for a run barefoot in the snow or maybe you read about his 28-hour climb to the snowy peak of Mt. Kilimanjaro, wearing nothing but a pair of running shorts and sneakers. That's what Wim does. It's part of his personal development philosophy...and it's teachable.

When I first discovered Wim I quickly became a fan. He was breaking a lot of what I thought were "the rules". I started to read all of his books and the various articles written about him. I watched video after video consuming as much as I could. I remember hearing him once say that anyone can do what he does, they just have to learn his method—the Wim Hoff Method. But I wasn't so sure about that.

I've always been attracted to vitality. Like so many of us, I have an inner desire pushing me to try and improve mentally, physically and spiritually. That quest led me to hire a U.S. Navy SEAL to live with me for a month. I also decided to run 100 miles within 24 hours to see how far I could push my limits. I managed to raise millions of dollars for charity in the process, but it was more than that for me. The run was something I was told couldn't be done—by me anyway. I knew the only way to prove the naysayers wrong was by testing my own self-imposed limits.

So the more I learned about Wim, the more I became intrigued. He had something that I wanted, but I wasn't sure what it was. I needed to find out. I eventually pulled the trigger and bought Wim's 10-week video seminar. I learned about his progressions of breathing/movement/yoga posture/meditative practices/cold exposure—and how it gave him a boost in certain physical and even spiritual markers. And then I bought a cold tub.

I set the temperature to 51 degrees and waited for the water to chill. The tub was intimidating as it gradually cooled down. The anticipation of submerging my body into the freezing water was messing with my mind...toying with me. The temperature dipped a degree every 15 minutes and each degree multiplied the fear. A few hours later it hit 51 degrees...it was GO time.

When I put my right foot in the water it took my breath away. Felt like I had been kicked in the gut by Nick Diaz. "Man, this is so damn cold", I thought. "Breathe", I told myself. "Just get your balls below this damn water, Jesse and you will be fine". As the water reached my belly button I exhaled deeply and relaxed my shoulders. I slowly lowered myself until the water hit my chin. An eerie calmness filled my spirit. I eased into the water. I felt alive.

Inspiration inspires. What I like most about Wim and his book is how he taught me to trust my body, overcome fear and give me the best opportunity for success. He mixes personal experience and science—which becomes truly motivating. Wim provides the tools you need to master self-discipline, gain courage and live a vibrant life. He is Aquaman and Tony Robbins rolled into one. He is The Iceman!

—**Jesse Itzler**
Author of **Living with a SEAL**

FOREWORD TO THE ENGLISH EDITION

BY MARTY GALLAGHER

Torpor is used to describe animal hibernation. When applied to humans, the word indicates a physiological and/or psychological sluggishness, a slowness or dull complacency. Affluence engenders torpor. Our soft modern lives lull us into complacent grooves. Our relatives in the not-too-distant past made their livings in highly physical occupations; nowadays we make our livings with our minds. Our physical side is so neglected and our occupations so devoid of any physicality that we invent gyms and fitness and diet plans to replace ploughing fields and running after game with a ferocity born out of hunger. As a species we are regressing; the body becomes less and less important. We live comfortable lives that require a minimum of physicality.

Weakness is the genesis of frailty, obesity, sickness and disease. We are weak. We are stuck in our respective warm wombs of sluggish complacency. We live virtual reality lives where everyone is a star in their own reality TV show; the Facebook mentality exaggerates our feelings of self-importance and provides our empty lives with a false sense of worth. Mired in the muck of torpor, we need to be jerked out of the sludge. Well, I found the man to do the jerking.

Henri Troyat once said of Count Leo Tolstoy, "He swaggered through life with his eyes wide open, his nostrils flared and his ears pricked." Wim Hof's method offers a way in which to access this type of electric, hypersensitive aliveness, a primal mindset that cannot be mentally conjured or purchased. Wim offers a way in which anyone can access the wonderment of the instantaneous present.

As an athlete and coach, I have spent a lifetime pondering how best to recalibrate the mind to improve human performance. High-level athletics, national and international level, requires a focus and concentration normal people can never experience or relate to—they have no frame of reference. Mind and body must unify to generate maximum athletic performance. A phenomenon all serious athletes have experienced is the way in which truly intense physical exercise alters the athlete's state-of-mind. After an intense training session, the elite athlete basks in an afterglow of pure bliss and contentment.

My postulate is that intense physical exercise offers a way in which to fold inner space, to access advanced levels of consciousness—the type, kind and flavour of consciousness that is sought after and experienced by advanced meditators.

Intense exercise short circuits the conscious mind, allowing the athlete to (unknowingly) attain advanced states of meditational consciousness. This higher state of consciousness is an unintended consequence of the intense training. The key to routinely accessing this bliss state is to present ourselves with a physical task of such severity that only by unifying body and mind can we succeed.

To successfully meld mind and body requires that the chattering mind, the internal commentator, cease its eternal yammering. We cannot generate the requisite 102% effort needed to succeed if we have even a hint of preoccupation. The elite athlete routinely subjects themselves to tasks so Herculean that only by achieving true and complete mind/body unification can they succeed with the task at hand.

The elite athlete methodically and consistently seeks to exceed their current capacities and limits. Only by continually assaulting the barricades of the status quo can the athlete hope to improve those limits and capacities. No athlete improves by striving to stay the same.

After fifty years of intense physical training, I can effortlessly access this "Mind of no Mind" via intense physical exercise. I can invoke a true and pristine mental silence in every workout. As an athletic monk and mystic, I can say with zero hesitation, I am at my best, as a person and as a man, as long as I remain enveloped in this exercise-induced state of altered consciousness. It is physiological and psychological Nirvana—addictive and exhilarating.

Over the interceding decades, my challenge has become: once attained, how can I extend my stay in this blissful, centered "glow state?" Once I enter this Nirvana of electric quietude, what can I do to extend my stay? I am still working on this: my current strategy is to roll from one "absorptive" task to the next: training to writing to cooking to running in the woods to music to careful reading...one creative task after another—then pass out at night in a regenerative sleep coma. Wake and repeat.

When the chattering monkey-mind comes back online, the bliss ends. Conscious thought is overrated. Krishnamurti nailed it: "The cessation of thought is the awakening of intelligence." Only when the ceaseless internal chatterbox is bitch-slapped into silence can we experience *reality*—reality always unfolds in the immediacy of the instantaneous present. Reality is like standing knee-deep in a raging stream. Only that is your life rushing by...

If you are thinking, you cannot perceive the immediate present, simple as that. Conscious thought exudes an inky film that blurs the perception of reality. The paradox is that one cannot use the conscious mind to silence the conscious mind; that would be just another expression of willpower and a form of suppression: an enforced mental silence is no silence at all. At some point the clenched fist must unclench.

Wim Hof has a far less complex way in which to access the bliss of the instantaneous present. Exposure to cold has the power to transport you into a wondrous state of higher consciousness. Mind and body *must* morph and meld in order to cope with the Herculean tasks Wim presents you with.

My entranceway requires equipment and great expertise and extreme exertion and time. Wim's method allows anyone to access the perfect present in a faster and simpler manner.

Wim has a specific definition for the concept of *commitment,* as it relates to his approach. If I were to be so bold, I would like to paraphrase his definition and relate it to my world. A person can stand ankle-deep in a freezing lake for the next 20 years and think they are doing something—and to a certain degree they are—the ankle wader is certainly better off than those that won't venture even this far. However, to reap the optimal physiological and psychological results, at some point the ankle wader must *take the plunge and commit!*

In my world, those that train at 70% of capacity attain 70% of their capacity. To commit, in my world, requires a man step up and handle 102% of capacity—consistently and repeatedly. The immediate gains and ongoing progress is attained by regularly and routinely and systematically exceeding current capacities. The elite powerlifter or elite spec ops fighter can routinely and regularly will themselves to operate past their capacity; no big deal at this level; strength of mind is one of the reasons why the elite are the elite.

Working at 102% in my world could be exemplified by a lifter in training setting a new personal record, pushing a 6th rep to lockout in the ultra-deep back squat with 635-pounds, one excruciating inch at a time with catastrophic physical collapse a real possibility. Yet still the elite push and struggle and embrace the pain. By locking out that 6th rep, by besting a previous best effort, maximum gains are reaped because the athlete maximally *committed*. That which does not kill me makes me stronger—and more muscular and far more rugged.

The ankle wader must, at some point, make the commitment and (literally) plunge into the extreme cold, embracing it fully and completely in order to absorb and realize the full and complete cornucopia of results. The 102% effort requires we push past the known, step off into the chasm. Dare to struggle, dare to win.

Most point to the *results* of Wim's method—the feats, the medical testing, the success of students, the reduction of disease and life-extending attributes—these are the results of Wim's method. I would respectfully point to the causes—I would suggest we look harder and with a greater sense of appreciation at the causes that power the Wim Hof Method.

You can fold inner space and experience the exhilaration of living in present-tense reality by submerging in an icy lake; this can be made into a meditational practice as profound and effective as sitting in deep Zazen in a Kyoto Monastery. The body-shocking severity of "The Cold—merciless and righteous," bitch-slaps the chattering mind into silence.

The breathing and the cold are the causes—the feats and tests and health benefits are the results. I would suggest that if you fall in love with the cause, results naturally and inevitably occur. In my world of Iron Zen, the ones that succeed are the ones that fall in love with the training, not the applause.

The breathing and the cold, the tools of the Wim Hof Method, will transport you, instantaneously, into the present, and an altered state of higher consciousness. The results you seek lie down the road—but in *every* Wim training session you have the opportunity to access the present and ergo, higher levels of consciousness. Is that not profound?

Wim's method induces psychological Nirvana. Wim's gateway method can be used by anyone—use it and quickly attain reality. Is this not monumental in and of itself? Use Wim's method to fold inner space. Join us and experience the exhilaration of living in the thought-free, super-sensitive, ultra-alert, stress-free present. The Samadhi state-of-being defines living with eyes wide open in the instantaneous present. Fall in love with the causes and results are inevitable.

— **Marty Gallagher**
  World champion team coach
  IPF world masters powerlifting champion
  *Author of **The Purposeful Primitive***

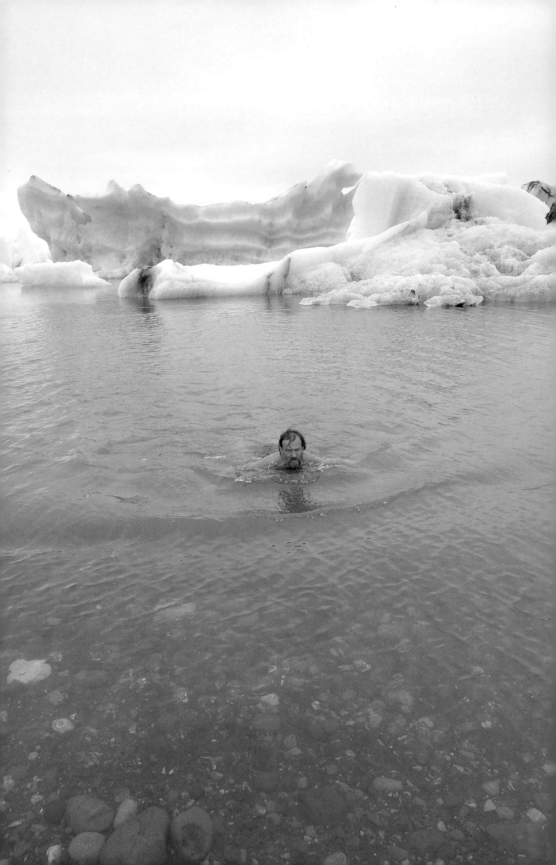

Prologue

By Koen de Jong

In October 2011, I watched a video clip on the internet of a man taking off his clothes and stepping into a lake—a cold lake somewhere in Iceland. The landscape was covered with snow and I saw icebergs. The clip was from a documentary by the BBC. The narrator said, "The water here is just above freezing, enough to kill most people within a minute."

But not this man.

He swam around calmly for fifteen minutes. "This guy is crazy," I thought to myself. But he also intrigued me. Who was he?

His name is Wim Hof.

Although I didn't immediately see the point in swimming around ice-floes, it aroused my curiosity. I watched another clip. This time, Hof swam *beneath* the ice. It got crazier, and I kept watching. Hof ran a marathon in the snow—bare-chested. He ran a half-marathon through the desert without drinking anything. He sat in a tank of ice for an hour and a quarter. He ran on Mount Everest in a pair of shorts.

After watching these clips for half an hour, I had one question: how was it possible?

Hof explained that 80% of what he does is related to breathing. Say, what? I've practiced breathing exercises for the past fifteen years and I've written a book about breathing, but there's no way I could swim under the ice without freezing to death.

Now I was even more curious.

What was Hof doing with his breathing methods that allowed him to accomplish so much more than anyone else? I really wanted to ask him about it in person. So I sent him an email through www. innerfire.nl. No one replied. I sent another one. No reply. Then I sent a third email and mentioned *Verademing*, the book on breathing that I wrote with Bram Bakker. Still no reply. But after six attempts, I finally got an answer. Enahm Hof, Wim's son explained, "It's very busy and so many people want to talk to Wim. They are conducting research at the Radboud University Medical Centre, which is taking up a lot of time."

Fortunately, I could drop by and talk to Wim.

We arranged to meet at an allotment in Amsterdam-West. Wim gave me a hearty greeting. He wore a T-shirt that said "No Rules Today". It's good to know that he not only defies the laws of physiology, but also rules in general.

The conversation was immediately pleasant and inspiring. During this first meeting, Wim explained a few breathing exercises and we did some right then and there. Surprisingly, it worked. I felt sharp and alert. He also explained that the cold training itself plays an important part in making you feel good. His extreme feats in the cold are not only a demonstration of what he can do with his body, the cold itself has a function. Hof is convinced that cold-training boosts health and has numerous rewards we can learn to take advantage of. He also told me how he discovered all this, and how he has helped people benefit substantially from his breathing exercises and the cold training.

Then I asked him why he performs all these extreme stunts.

His eyes widened as he said, "Our breathing is the link between the physical world and the soul. If we, as human beings, can find the way back to our souls, we will win the war."

Wim saw the astounded expression on my face and roared with laughter, adding, "I mean the war against bacteria and viruses."

His extreme feats are not an end in themselves. He wants to show what the human body is capable of—not just his body, but everyone's, including yours and mine. Wim is never sick. For many people, his methods work much better than medicine. But until recently, it was not clear exactly how his methods work. Now, there is good news: the secret Wim has known for decades has recently been confirmed by science.

We can influence our body's *autonomic nervous system*.

Wim's method was studied at the Radboud University Medical Centre in the Dutch city of Nijmegen. What does it mean for metabolic diseases like rheumatism and Crohn's disease? What does it mean for healthy people? How much extra energy can it give you? Wim can run marathons in the snow, but what are we—mere mortals—capable of? Can we use that energy in our work? Can we use Wim's methods to cure type II diabetes? It sounds almost too good to be true.

And yet, Wim wants his method to conquer the world. I am a willing guinea pig and have started with the breathing exercises. I

take cold ice baths and practice to strengthen my commitment—
and I've taken note of everything I've experienced. I've also spoken
to a lot of people who have started using Wim's method. This book
is a reflection of all these experiences, and of course the technique,
background, and the foundations of Wim's method.

I write mainly using the word "we", because this book has been
written on the basis of both our inputs. Wim has mostly contributed
the substantive knowledge. Every now and again, I will write in the
first person singular, because I want to observe Wim from a distance.
Now you know, "we" is Wim and Koen and "I" is me, Koen.

Enjoy reading this book—and good luck with the cold showers.

—Koen de Jong

INTRODUCTION

I n this book, we will describe a method that combines breathing exercises, cold training and commitment. The method is named after Wim Hof, as he is the one who brought these three components together. It is also named after Hof for practical reasons—he is already well-known for his many appearances on television showing what he can do with the cold.

The method is based on Wim Hof's many years of training in the natural environment. For a long time, he has tested the limits of his body by exposing it to increasingly extreme challenges. One important discovery he made during this process was the ability to control his bodily functions in a way that science had not deemed possible.

For example, anyone can lift up their right hand and scratch their nose with their index finger, but no one can fight bacteria that have been injected into their arm. Hof can do that. He can influence and control his autonomic nervous system. The autonomic nervous system regulates things like your body temperature, heart rate, blood pressure, breathing, and determines whether your blood vessels dilate or contract. In other words, everything that automatically happens in your body.

"Normal" people cannot control these functions. In the autonomic nervous system, everything happens automatically. The fact that Hof can control his autonomic functions has long been regarded as a medical wonder. But Hof sees it differently: he is convinced that everyone is theoretically capable of influencing their own autonomic nervous systems.

In 2014, he was proven correct. A scientific study conducted at the Radboud University Medical Centre with 24 test subjects showed that people who had practiced the Hof method were all able to control their autonomic nervous systems.

A Discovery That Will Change the World

It's impossible to predict the potentially far-reaching consequences of this discovery. If people can influence their autonomic nervous systems, what will that mean for those suffering from autoimmune diseases? Autoimmune diseases occur when the immune system attacks the body's own cells and tissue by mistake. If you are able to influence your own autonomic nervous system, can you let your body know that the autoimmune disease is harmful? And can people who are overweight tell their bodies to use their otherwise energy-depleting stored fats as fuel?

If we really can control our bodies, this opens up countless possibilities. So far we have only mentioned serious diseases, but according to Hof, his method can also be used to cure a normal hangover after a night out on the town. It can give you a lot more energy, even if you are perfectly healthy.

Now that Hof has scientifically proven he can influence his nervous system, he wants nothing more than to teach as many people as possible how to use his method. Although, when one woman asked what she would learn from one of his courses, he answered "I can't teach you anything, you're only here to learn *not* to do certain things."

Hof was referring to tapping into the physical capacity already in our bodies. We just have to find the key to rediscover that physical potential. To do that, you only need to do two things: breathing exercises and cold training. To do these two things properly, you will need to make a resolute commitment. These three components—breathing exercises, cold training and commitment—constitute what we call the Wim Hof Method (WHM).

We will describe these three components in three separate chapters, and of course give you exercises that you can do at home. You can start immediately, today.

We will also give you background information on the exercises. You will learn how to tell if the exercises are working and how they can affect you physiologically. Hof will share many of his experiences to inspire you and to give a deeper understanding of what happens when you use his method. But, he is an extremist. You don't have to go to Iceland to swim among the icebergs for a quarter of an hour. Taking cold showers is enough to start. For that reason, we will tell you about people who are already using the Wim Hof Method. Some of them have fascinating stories to tell. Marianne Peper, for example, used to take twelve different medications for her rheumatism. She was unable to dress herself because of the pain. Now she no longer takes any pills and feels very healthy.

We hope that stories like these will inspire you to start doing the exercises. Just the combination of breathing exercises and cold training can produce startling results. We understand that you may be skeptical and won't take our enthusiastic stories at face value. But, if you are skeptical, you are also curious and inquiring.

Hof also has critics who are not skeptical, but cynical. They call him a charlatan. When skepticism turns into cynicism, it is harder to see what works and what is possible. So, please read this book with a healthy dose of skepticism, but don't allow yourself to become too cynical.

Before we learn about cold training, let's first take a closer look at Wim Hof. Who is this man, and why can he do so much more than other people?

WIM HOF

Because Wim Hof's method carries his name, we want to tell you a little about him before you start working with the WHM. It's important to know how he decided to seek out the cold and why he became increasingly extreme in that quest.

SITTARD

Wim Hof was born in the southern Dutch town of Sittard in 1959. He had seven brothers and two sisters. He was born in the corridor of the hospital. After his mother had given birth to his twin brother André, no one noticed that a second child was on the way. When the doctors had left, his mother started to feel contractions coming on again.

His mother, a Catholic, prayed that the second child would also be born healthy. She expressed the hope that if it were healthy, the child would grow up to be a missionary. Wim's mother told this story regularly and Wim believed the circumstances of his birth and his mother's strength had a great influence on him in his younger years.

Hof was fascinated by the cold from a very early age. One freezing winter's night when he was seven, a neighbor found him in the snow. Strongly attracted by the white landscape, Hof had climbed out of bed, crept outside, and fallen asleep in the snow. If his neighbor had not discovered him, he probably would have frozen to death.

As a young boy, Hof also loved books. At the age of nine, he was already reading books on exotic religions, yoga and meditation. His interest was sparked by his older brother, who had spent several months hitchhiking around the Middle and Far East and had come back with strange and wonderful tales. Forty years ago, a journey through Turkey, Iran, Pakistan and India was still shrouded in mystery.

His brother had changed, not only on the inside, but also in his appearance. His hair and his clothes made him very conspicuous on the street. Wim looked up to his brother and felt strongly attracted to faraway lands and strange religions. He also noticed an energy and cheerfulness in his brother that made him curious.

While still very young, Hof learned to meditate from books on Hinduism and Buddhism in the local library. In the Catholic church in Sittard, he would concentrate on his breathing rather than listen to the sermon. When he was only ten years old, Hof taught himself yoga from the book *Yoga, Immortality and Freedom*, by Mircea Eliade. He went to school with a healthy reluctance and was known as a self-willed, clever and cheerful young boy.

He had a strong desire to learn—not at an intellectual level, but by experiencing things himself.

At the age of 17, Wim decided to leave school and travel to India. He wanted to find a teacher who knew more about what is really important in life. He was looking for a deeper spiritual understanding.

INDIA—COLD WATER IN THE GANGES

He flew to Karachi and took the train to New Delhi. In search of yogis, he slept in the enormous Birla Mandir temple complex. He met the owner of a teahouse and the rebellious son of a carpet magnate there. These two men persuaded Hof to accompany them to Rishikesh and Badrinath, two places of pilgrimage on the Ganges.

This colorful trio set off together: a strong, bearded Sikh who ran a teahouse, a black sheep from the carpet industry who could get anything he wanted—and who was fed up with the corruption of his world—and Hof. They thought Hof was crazy because he went swimming in the Ganges a couple of times a day. Hof even swam across to the other side, no mean feat given the strong current. He also impressed them with the acrobatic yoga exercises he could do, despite never having had a yoga lesson in his life.

In India, Hof discovered that his autodidactic approach had already brought him a long way. He could already stand on one leg and put the other behind his neck, a position many people have to practice for years to master.

His traveling companions remained behind in an ashram, but Hof didn't feel at home there. He didn't like the "clingy-cozy" atmosphere of the foreign participants, and although many of the yogis had learned very special techniques, he didn't like the way they profited from them. He also discovered that he could not learn much from them, as he had already mastered their tricks. He continued his travels alone on foot.

COLD WATER—A DISCOVERY

In a spot where the Ganges crashes down between sky-high mountains in a cascade of waterfalls, Hof had a wondrous experience. He felt inner peace and enormous strength. He had an irresistible urge to jump into the dangerous waterfall—and did just that. After a difficult swim, Hof stood under the mighty waterfall. His thoughts were immediately cut off by the cold water.

The sensation of a strength and power much greater than himself took hold of him. Since then, he has loved ice-cold water.

So Hof traveled to India—the cradle of spirituality—in search of noumenon (the spirit behind the esoteric books) and discovered the impact cold had on his body and above all, his mind.

After this discovery, Hof did not stay in India much longer. He loved the country, the climate, and the people, but he missed the Netherlands and decided to go back home. He did not know what he was going to do yet, but the lesson of the ice-cold water had made a deep impression on him. He knew he had to do something with it.

AMSTERDAM

Hof went to live in a squat in Amsterdam in 1979 at the age of 20. Through one of his brother's friends, he got a place in De Wielingen, an old orphanage, where he lived with ninety other squatters. He led an ascetic life, eating little and doing a lot of yoga. His lifestyle was very different from that of the hippy-like students in the squat. They used LSD, smoked joints, and ate space-cake to achieve altered states of consciousness.

In the Vondelpark, Hof shared the yoga positions he had mastered with anyone who was interested. He also liked to explain their physiological basis. One sunny autumn day, Hof was swimming in the pond in the park. Soaking wet, he sat down in the sun to dry. Then he felt two hands on his back, which began to massage him. Hof remained sitting in his yoga position. He did not look up or around, but there, in the open-air theatre in the Vondelpark, he felt love. After the massage, he turned around, and looked straight into the eyes of the woman who massaged him. She made him beam with joy.

The woman's name was Olaya. She was Spanish—or, more precisely, Basque. From that moment in the park, they were inseparable for a year. Deeply in love, Olaya moved in with Hof at the squat. For that first year, they did not have sex, even though they slept together on a single sleeping mat. Their platonic relationship was warm and physical. Hof's life was devoted to yoga, and his Spanish girlfriend respected that.

After a year, Olaya got homesick and returned to her family home in Northern Spain. Hof wanted to see more of the world, so he and his twin brother cycled to Senegal.

A CITY BIKE TO SENEGAL

The two brothers set out for Senegal from Sittard on two regular city bikes. During this journey, Hof discovered how the sun affected his mood. Although the two brothers left in the autumn, the sun shone incessantly. Bad memories and depressive thoughts disappeared during their daily rides in the sun. Hof regularly thought of how Vincent van Gogh suffered less from depression in the South of France. Once again, Hof experienced the great impact of a "normal" natural phenomenon.

During the bike journey, Hof also had a deep spiritual experience, in which his body and mind became one. The sense of duality seemed to have disappeared—a new breakthrough for Hof. His body was now a vehicle, not just a tool. He had this feeling one morning, after an intense period of yoga training. Around that same time, the brothers met Wolfgang, a friendly German they caught up with in the Pyrenees. Wolfgang wanted to learn yoga from Wim. Because Wolfgang was on his way to Algiers, and not Senegal, the lessons were very fast and intensive. Wim explained the physiological effects of yoga, and taught Wolfgang many of his skills. The profundity they achieved in their practice proved to be another important step forward for Wim.

After this illuminating cycling trip, Hof went back to India. This time, he searched for the power of nature, not for yogis. He trained his body and mind under extreme circumstances. Sometimes he spent several days at great heights while enduring temperatures of -2°C (28.4°F), without food. He discovered a new way to survive the extreme cold: controlling his breathing. With breathing exercises, he could transform his fear and the negative experience of the cold into a powerful form of energy. He saw his body in a new way, and learned that breathing is an important instrument. This was also where he learned his breathing exercises.

A MESSAGE TO THE READER

We want to put your mind at ease. You're probably asking yourself, "I wanted to read a book about the cold and hard science. So what's all this about spirituality, yoga, duality, and ashrams?" Don't worry, all that will be explained in great detail in the coming chapters. But, now that science has embraced Hof's method, it is important to know where his knowledge originated. You won't need to go to India and sit on a cold mountain in some impossible yoga position.

Before we continue with the cold, we first must share the sad story of Wim's wife, Olaya.

OLAYA

Before Hof went to India for the second time, he returned to Amsterdam. He missed Olaya and they met each other again in the city. After two years apart, the love between them was as strong as ever. They got married. In 1983, they had a son, Enahm. The proud parents rented a house and two daughters followed, Isabelle (1985) and Laura (1986).

But, Olaya found the cold climate of the Netherlands difficult. Eventually, the family of five emigrated to the warm side of the Pyrenees. Wim found work teaching English, and they rented a farmhouse just outside Estella. They dreamed of setting up a center where creative individuals could come together and learn yoga, philosophy, or painting—and where you could walk for hours.

Hof was happy, but still restless and searching for new challenges. This led him to do a lot of mountain-climbing. One day, he climbed a steep rock face with only a hemp rope, a small hammer and a few pitons. Olaya was furious that he was willing to risk his life climbing in that way, since they had three children. Hof had an uncontrollable urge to climb, but also felt responsible for his wife and children.

He decided to stop climbing, and to control his urge to climb, he developed a breathing technique that allowed him to stay underwater for more than six minutes. Every morning, he went to a nearby lake to meditate and practice staying underwater.

But the tension between Hof and his wife remained. One day, she disappeared and did not return for several months. Olaya suffered from attacks of rage and depression, and expressed her unhappiness by regularly threatening to take her own life. But she refused to seek treatment. The family returned to Amsterdam because the remote farmhouse no longer felt safe.

Back in Amsterdam, their youngest son Michael was born in 1998. Shortly after the birth, Olaya left again, without saying anything. Her depression was very difficult for her and it was a tough time for Hof, too.

When he contacted Olaya, he never knew what her mood would be in advance. Sometimes, she spent three or four months with Hof and their children, but then she would spend three or four months at her parents' house. In the summer, Wim worked as a climbing trip group leader, and the family of six all stayed with Olaya's parents in Pamplona.

Hof had a good relationship with Olaya's Spanish family and friends. He learned about the culture and how to speak Basque. He did his best to be a good father and son-in-law, but he still needed moments to challenge himself in silence, away from the daily routine. He saw that Olaya would sometimes sit and stare straight forward strangely, but he did not really respond to it. And she continued to refuse treatment for her increasingly severe depression. Sometimes, she would slap someone hard in the face for no reason. She loved her children, but announced that she wanted to divorce Wim. He did not know if she had said this "only" for attention. He felt powerless and started climbing again to keep from losing himself.

One day, when Hof was alone in the mountains, Olaya jumped from the eighth floor of her parents' house in Pamplona.

Olaya was dead. Enahm, Isabelle, Laura, and Michael lost their mother, and Wim lost his wife. He felt guilty and the children were devastated.

Hof devoted himself to caring for his children, occasionally retreating to be alone with nature to re-charge his batteries. In those years, he was a well-known figure in the Vondelpark. With ropes and belay equipment, he showed young children how to climb the highest trees. The children learned that they could do more than they thought was possible. Hof enjoyed the natural surroundings, even in the heart of Amsterdam.

Later, Wim remarried and had another son.

INNERFIRE

The children grew up and Hof looked for new challenges. His breathing techniques, yoga and cold training gave him enormous strength—and he liked to share it with others. The media got him in their sights. Encouraged by the attention and the effect it had on other people, Wim broke record after record. He took the longest bath in ice. He climbed snow-covered mountain peaks, wearing shorts. He ran a marathon in Lapland at -30°C (-22°F). He swam hundreds of meters under the ice.

These records earned him the nickname "The Iceman".

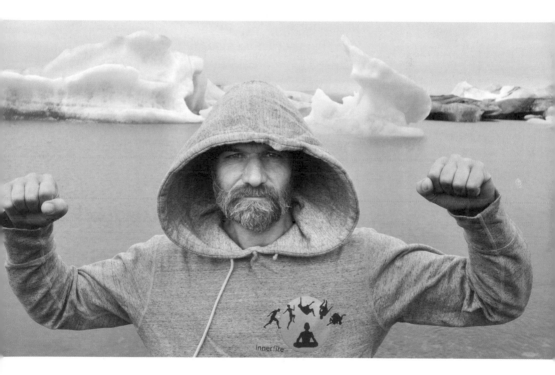

His records were reported on television in Japan, Germany, Poland, Spain and many other countries. The BBC made a documentary about him, and millions of people watched his feats on the internet.

Hof enjoyed the attention and the expanding potentialities of his body. But, something started to gnaw at him. Perhaps because he was getting older—or because of his five children. Or, maybe he was still coming to terms with Olaya's suicide.

He felt the need to share his knowledge and the possibilities of his body with more people. Could other people do what he can do? In 2007, the renowned Feinstein Institute in New York studied Hof. The results showed that he was able to control his autonomic nervous system. For Wim, the results were logical—after all, he had trained to do it for many years. But, the researchers thought he was a medical wonder.

From then on, Hof put himself at the disposal of science. His main aim was to show others that they could also train to do what he does. It was the start of a very special time in Wim's life. He attracted more and more attention and those who started using his method were wildly enthusiastic.

In 2010, Hof's eldest son Enahm set up a company called Innerfire. The combination of breathing exercises and cold training had far-reaching effects on people over and over again. They started organizing workshops and trips, and the method was increasingly validated by science. In the Netherlands, more and more people learned to train others in the Wim Hof Method (WHM). In the near future, people will be able to learn the method, under supervision, in many places around the country.

Hof's daughter, Isabelle and his son Michael now both work at Innerfire.

More and more people are using Wim's techniques, including leading Dutch entertainer Theo Maassen, former Minister of Finance Gerrit Zalm, athletes, people with rheumatism and Crohn's disease, psychiatrists, cardiologists and internists. Companies ask Hof to sit in ice baths with hundreds of managers at a time.

At the same time, more researchers are now studying the WHM at the Radboud University Medical Centre, the Amsterdam Medical Centre, and at universities in Boston and New York.

Why is that?

What is the secret of Wim Hof's method?

That is what we are going to tell you, starting with cold training.

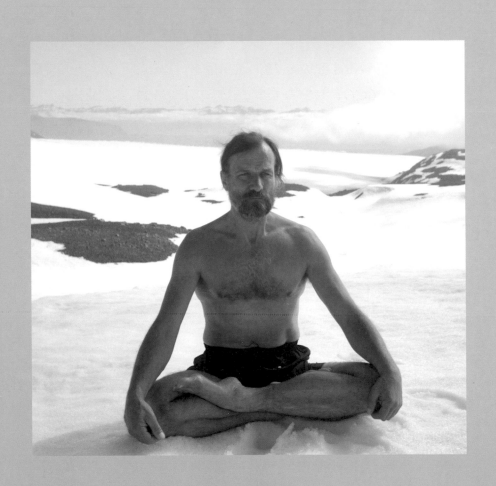

COLD TRAINING

"You can't learn anything from the cold.
But you can learn to not do some things."
—Wim Hof

We are addicted to temperatures around 20-21°C (68-71°F). In the summer, we switch on the air-conditioning in the car, and in the winter we set the central heating to about 20°C (68°F). Companies and shops do the same, so we spend much of our time in roughly the same temperatures. Double glazing, insulation, and concrete all help us to maintain the temperatures we like. In the winter, we wear coats, scarves, hats, gloves and thick socks to make it easier for our bodies. This feels comfortable and pleasant.

We have gotten used to it.

That is a pity. In the winter, we can actually use the cold, rather than continually protect ourselves from it. Exposure to cold has a favorable effect on our health and our moods. In some parts of Scandinavia, Russia, and China, ice-hole swimming is popular. The swimmers saw a hole in the ice and immerse themselves in water that is just above the freezing point.

Cold is considered to have many benefits. It is supposedly good for:

- Circulation
- The heart
- Glossy hair
- Taut skin
- Increased energy levels
- Improved mood
- Fighting infections
- Self-confidence

But, what happens to you when you get cold? How can exposure to cold be so beneficial?

Your body has 125,000 km (77,671 miles) of blood vessels. If you laid them end to end, they would go around the world three times. All these blood vessels ensure that the billions of cells in your body continually get enough nutrients and oxygen. If they work properly, your whole body will function better, because it will get more nutrients and oxygen. Your brain will work better and the same applies to your muscles, intestines, heart, liver and so on.

WHAT ELSE DO WE KNOW ABOUT BLOOD VESSELS?

When you measure or feel your pulse, you are sensing the heart beat through your arteries. One of the best known arteries is the aorta, which connects your heart to the other arteries. The coronary artery makes sure that the heart muscle is supplied with blood. Your head and your brain receive blood through the cerebral arteries. Blood vessels divide and supply your whole body with blood. Smaller blood vessels called capillaries, are very narrow. Oxygen and nutrients are filtered through the thin capillary walls to your tissue cells. Blood that is low in oxygen returns to your heart through the veins.

Blood is transported from the intestines by the portal vein to the liver, where harmful substances are removed as much as possible.

This gigantic web of arteries and veins is crucial to many functions in your body. If your blood vessels are open and working properly, your whole body will benefit.

What does all this have to do with cold?

When you expose yourself to the cold, by stepping into a cold lake for example, your body automatically closes off blood flow to the less vital parts of your body. That is necessary because your body temperature must not fall below 35°C (95°F). It is more important that your heart keeps beating than that your little toe gets enough blood. Your body is smart enough to give priority to your heart and your other vital organs. Your arms and legs get less blood as their blood vessels contract. This ensures that your vital organs—your heart, liver, lungs and kidneys—get enough blood to continue working. Your arms and legs will start to tingle and you might feel a burning sensation. When the body warms up again, the blood vessels open up and your circulation normalizes.

By exposing your body to the cold, you can train your blood vessels by closing them forcefully, then making them open again. It's like training your muscles. For example, you can train weak arm muscles by doing push-ups. At first, your muscles will hurt and feel weaker. But after they have recovered, they are stronger. It's the same with your blood vessels. You benefit from having stronger arms even when you are not doing push-ups in the same way that you will also benefit from having open blood vessels when you are not cold. But you can train your blood vessels by exposing them to the cold.

People who regularly train in the cold say (almost without exception) that they feel the cold less. We hear time and time again about the energy "boost" they get from the cold, and how it affects their mood. But, despite all its benefits, cold is also a dangerous force. You can achieve a lot if you build up your exposure slowly, but if you go too fast, it can be dangerous.

COLD DAMAGE

If you expose yourself to extreme cold for too long without training, you run the risk of suffering cold damage. If your core body temperature falls below 35°C (95°F), the cold will get into your bones and tissues can die. That is what happens when people get frostbite on their fingers and toes while climbing in the Himalayas or other high mountain ranges. First, the fingers or toes become white, which is accompanied by a burning or tingling sensation. After a while, they become completely numb, which is dangerous. If they are not treated, the skin will become dark or even black. The skin will look as if it had been burnt.

Of course, hypothermia (when the core body temperature falls below 35°C) doesn't just affect the toes and fingers. Your normal metabolic functions are also at risk: your heart rate and blood pressure lower and your breathing slows down. Eventually, you will lose consciousness and after an hour, it will be fatal. In ice water, this process happens even more quickly to untrained people. In water, the cold can be fatal after only half an hour.

Wim Hof can sit in a tank full of ice for an hour and a half while his body temperature remains constant at 37°C (98.6°F). His heart rate and blood pressure remain normal, too.

HOW IS THIS PHYSICALLY POSSIBLE?

Research by Hopman et al. (2010) shows that when exposed to ice, Hof's metabolic rate increases by 300%. This also increases his body's heat production. According to Hopman, Hof can turn up his

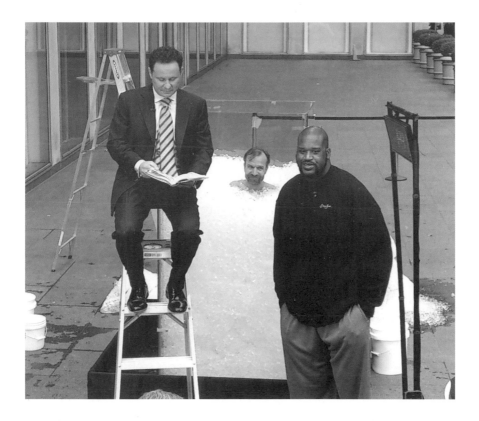

body's "stove" three times higher than normal. Most people will start to shiver and shake to stay warm, but Hof doesn't do that either. He stays warm by controlling his autonomic nervous system with breathing exercises just before the cold exposure. Hof's training has given him a lot of brown fat, which means he stays warm more easily.

There are two varieties of fat:

- **White fat**
- **Brown fat**

White fat mainly stores energy and is a reserve of nutrients. Beneath the skin, it serves as insulation for your body. It protects your organs, and also ensures that they stay in place.

The main function of brown fat is warming up your body by burning fatty acids and glucose.

One consequence of Hof's many years of training is that he has a lot of brown fat. Brown fat releases energy directly, generating heat. Newborn babies have a lot of brown fat, so that they can warm up quickly in a cold environment. After nine months, there is little left of this brown fat. Each year, it decreases, perhaps because of clothes and blankets. Adults in Western societies have almost no brown fat left.

It now appears that brown fat tissue can be activated by cold (from Marken-Lichtenbeld et al. 2011). It starts to be stimulated at 18°C (64.4°F) when fatty acids are activated to keep the body at the right temperature. The lower the temperature, the more brown fat tissue is activated. In a room at 11°C (51.8°F), Hof produces 35% more body heat than at normal room temperature—thanks to his brown fat. His body heat increases up to 50%, while young adults only produce 20% more body heat at the same temperature.

People who are overweight (which is always excess white fat) who train in the cold, can teach their bodies to turn the white fat into fuel via brown fat.

The benefits of cold training are not just restricted to blood vessels and brown fat, but extend to the production of white corpuscles.

WHITE CORPUSCLES

You have between five and six liters (1.3-1.6 gallons) of blood flowing through your body. Blood consists of 55% plasma and 45% corpuscles. Plasma is mainly water with minerals, carbohydrates, fats, hormones and more than 100 different kinds of protein.

There are three types of corpuscles: blood platelets (thrombocytes), red corpuscles (erythrocytes) and white corpuscles (leukocytes). Platelets help heal wounds by ensuring that the blood stops flowing and a scab forms. Red corpuscles absorb oxygen in the lungs and transport it to the organs. The red corpuscle cells contain hemoglobin, which gives blood its red color and binds with oxygen. White corpuscles are a collective name for different cells. They are larger than red corpuscles and you have fewer of them. They defend the body against infection from bacteria, viruses, parasites, fungi, yeasts, and foreign substances. If we have an infection, we also have more white corpuscles, since the body will produce them to fight it.

Research carried out by the Thrombosis Foundation (Documentation Centre 1994) shows that people who take a cold shower daily also have more white corpuscles. The researchers explain the increase in white corpuscles by the activation of the immune system, which releases more white corpuscles.

The great advantage of knowing about brown and white fat, and red and white corpuscles is that you will know at least a little about what happens to your body when you are exposed to cold. That can encourage you to train yourself to withstand cold. Cold training can affect a lot of physical complaints including excess weight, fungi, and viruses—along with helping to open up lax blood vessels. But even without this knowledge, you will notice that something happens to you if you take cold showers or get into an ice bath.

On the first of January, 2015, more than 3,000 people started taking cold showers as part of the "Cool Challenge". One initiator of the challenge was Dr. Geert Buijze of the Amsterdam Medical Centre. Wim Hof clearly experiences effects from exposure to extreme cold in combination with breathing exercises, but Buijze was curious to know whether just taking cold showers had any effect. During the challenge, it was remarkable how quickly many people got used to the cold and started to feel the benefits after only three or four showers. Many said that after showering, their skin quickly turned red—a sign of good blood circulation. For more of their experiences and the results of the study, see www.coolchallenge.nl.

Profile of Jack Egberts, who worked with the WHM.

JACK EGBERTS (1971)

Jack Egberts is a lawyer in Leeuwarden, in the northern Dutch province of Friesland. He had been tired and listless for some time. He had always been active and energetic, but he was diagnosed with Lyme disease. The doctors who diagnosed the disease could do little for him. But Egberts did not accept that there was nothing he could do, and looked for alternatives on the internet. After searching for "more energy", he found Wim Hof. He was immediately curious and wanted to know more.

Egberts has a large and successful law firm. He never does anything half-way. So when he found Wim, he didn't sign up for just one day, he signed up for a whole week. The favorable effects of the cold training were enormous. After a week of "Hoffing", as he calls it, Egberts hardly had any trouble from the Lyme disease. Better than that, he now had more energy than before the disease. Everything changed, his energy, eating habits, and all the symptoms of Lyme disease disappeared.

At first, Egberts had a lot of reservations because it all seemed too good to be true. He is still a down-to-earth Frisian and a well-read lawyer—rationality rules. And yet, he was soon unable to keep his enthusiasm about the results of the training to himself. He persuaded his mother to take cold showers. She has been taking medication for high blood pressure for years. As Egberts told the story, he had a broad grin on his face: after one month, she had no more symptoms and could stop taking the medication. Completely.

Profiles like this will appear regularly in *The Way of The Iceman*. Of course, they are only intended as information and to inspire you. They are not intended to encourage you to stop taking medication or end a course of treatment without first consulting your doctor.

Would you like to know how to achieve these benefits, for your own enhanced well-being?

Below are a few exercises for you to try out.

DO-IT-YOURSELF: TAKING COLD SHOWERS

Take a warm shower, as you always do. Then, while the water is still warm, start doing the following breathing exercises: Breathe in and breathe out slowly. Breathe in deeply and breathe out nice and slow. Keep doing this for about a minute—taking a total of six to ten breaths. Then, turn the shower to cold.

Of course, you will start breathing more quickly and the cold will give you a shock. The trick is to breathe calmly again. Control your breathing under the cold shower. The moment your breathing is under control, the cold will feel different. If you find it difficult to set the shower to cold in one go, do it in two or three steps. You can also start by just holding your feet under the cold spray, then your hands and arms, then gradually bringing your whole body under the cold shower.

Stay under the cold shower for a minute.

If you are unable to relax with the breathing exercise, try another trick—rubbing yourself. You can "lead" the cold spray over your body with your hands. Massage your arms and legs as the cold water goes over them. The cold might feel a little less intense.

DO-IT-YOURSELF: A BOWL OF ICE-COLD WATER

Fill a bucket or bowl with cold water. Add some ice (you can make ice by putting plastic containers filled with water in the freezer). Put your hands in the cold water. At first, it will tingle painfully, as the blood vessels contract. But the pain will quickly decrease, and when you feel your hands becoming warm, you can stop. It sounds crazy that your hands will feel warm from being in ice-cold water, but it really happens, because your body "turns up the thermostat". If your hands are not warm after two minutes, you can stop.

How can your hands become warm while they are in ice-cold water?

Wim calls it "collateral smear", a phenomenon caused by a hormone that makes the walls of your blood vessels strong and elastic. When you immerse parts of your body in cold water, it releases strengthening hormones and an anti-freeze hormone. These hormones ensure that the vascular system continues to work automatically.

Cold showers and a bowl of cold water with ice in it are excellent starter exercises. We recommend that you try it for a month. After that month, you can continue with your cold training. In the winter, you can swim outside. Wouldn't it be fantastic if in a couple of years time, people started swimming in the canals of Amsterdam en masse in the winter? While I was writing this book, I became so enthusiastic about cold training that I went swimming in the Admiralengracht canal in Amsterdam in December during a light frost. After a few times, I got more and more reactions from people. Half of them were curious and we had fascinating conversations about the cold, health and illnesses. Others thought I was mentally ill and should be protected from myself. Someone called the police and I had to explain why I was swimming in the canal. After I explained that I was writing this book about cold training, they let me go home to warm up. This shows how new and unusual it all is. Many of my friends thought swimming in the canal was stupid and that the water was dirty. I thought that it wouldn't be that bad—after all, Princess Máxima had also swam in the canals during the Amsterdam City Swim, to collect money for research into lesser known diseases; in 2014, that was amyotrophic lateral sclerosis (ALS). If they even let the princess—now the Queen—swim in the canal, then it couldn't be that dangerous.

Anyway, before you saw a hole in the ice and plunge into the cold water, start by taking cold showers and doing the breathing exercises.

Summary

- Exposure to cold improves your circulation
- Exposure to cold activates brown fat tissue
- Exposure to cold activates the production of white corpuscles
- Do-it-yourself: take cold showers
- Do-it-yourself: immerse your hands and feet in a bowl of ice water

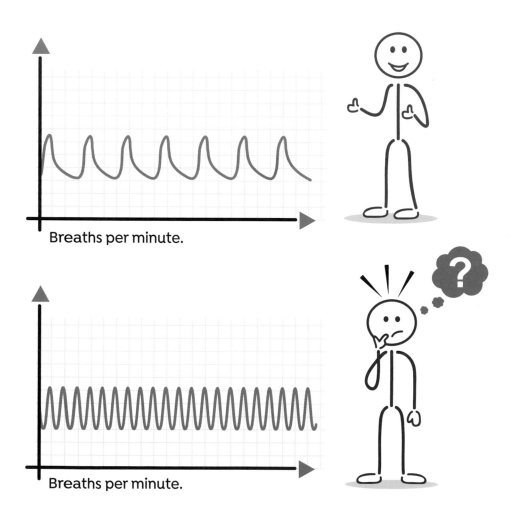

Breaths per minute.

Breaths per minute.

BREATHING

"It's not hocus pocus, it's physiology."
—Wim Hof

We started the chapter on cold with the assumption that you prefer temperatures of around 20-21°C (68-70°F). We explained how cold can have a positive effect on your mood and your health. There is a good chance that you have become accustomed to breathing in a certain way—and that can be improved, too.

Many people breathe 13, 15, 17, 20 or as many as 22 or more times a minute. Even when they are sitting quietly in a chair, reading a book. A resting respiratory rate of between six and ten times a minute is enough. Is it bad if you breathe faster than that? Yes, it can be—and we explain why below.

Breathing exercises are considered to have many benefits. They can:

- Help you relax
- Give you more energy
- Help you sleep better
- Help relieve headaches
- Are good for extreme athletes
- Help relieve back and neck problems
- Help relieve intestinal problems

Before we tell you more about the physiology of breathing, first take a look at how you are breathing right now.

DO-IT-YOURSELF:
CHECK YOUR OWN RESPIRATORY RATE

Count how often you breathe in a minute. Each breath begins as you start to breathe in and ends when you stop exhaling, just before you inhale again. Count how often you breathe in 60 seconds and you will know your respiratory rate at this moment.

Just by counting your breaths, you will probably start breathing differently, simply because you are paying attention. So it won't be a completely accurate picture of how you were breathing before you started to count, but it will give you an idea.

If you breathe more than ten times a minute, then your body is ready for action, but your respiratory rate is not compatible with sitting quietly. Imagine sitting on a chair while you are breathing about 18 times a minute—you would be breathing as though you are running through the park. Of course, you can't keep that up all day— never mind weeks on end. People suffering from fatigue often look at the cyclists in the Tour de France in admiration and amazement. It's tough to cycle more than 150 km (93.2 miles) every day for three weeks. Yet, people who feel tired and have a high respiratory rate are working nearly as hard. When a competitive cyclist rests, he breathes only six times a minute and has a heart rate of less than 40 beats per minute. People who are tired breathe too quickly all day and mostly have a resting heart rate of 70 beats per minute or higher.

If a rapid respiratory rate becomes normal for you, you will start to develop health problems.

I have described the benefits of calm breathing earlier in, *Verademing*, a book I wrote with psychiatrist Bram Bakker. In that book, we showed how irregular breathing leads to health problems. Irregular breathing is either breathing too fast or deeper than necessary.

There is growing interest in correct breathing. More and more doctors and psychologists recommend practicing breath work to relax. Yoga, meditation and mindfulness are becoming increasingly popular. There is growing scientific evidence of the benefits of breathing exercises and meditation. Science is building a bridge between ancient meditation techniques and the much younger Western medicine.

BREATHING TECHNIQUES: BUTEYKO AND VAN DER POEL

There are many techniques for breathing besides meditation. The methods of Konstantin Buteyko and Stans van der Poel are very popular in the Netherlands. Buteyko (1923-2003) was a Ukrainian doctor who studied medicine in Moscow. He discovered the effect of breathing exercises on health on October 7, 1952. He had to diagnose a patient who was breathing heavily and who sometimes gasped for breath. Buteyko thought he was dealing with an anxious asthma patient. To his surprise, there were no signs of asthma, but the patient had high blood pressure.

Because Buteyko also suffered from high blood pressure, he started thinking. He observed that he also breathed deeply and heavily. So, he went to his surgery and tried to make his breathing as calm as possible. To his surprise, he noticed that his blood pressure decreased, and his headache faded away.

Buteyko started looking for other links between breathing and health problems. With a lot of practice, he even managed to get his blood pressure back to a normal range without medication. He used this experience to start helping his patients to breathe more calmly and less deeply. He noticed that asthma patients could stop attacks by continuing to breathe calmly.

At the end of the 1950s, Buteyko had his own laboratory fitted out with modern equipment, and he was put in charge of a team of medical specialists. The time was ripe to study the link between breathing and a wide variety of chemical processes in the body and several diseases from a scientific perspective. Buteyko's research showed that deep, fast breathing can cause a variety of health problems, including high blood pressure, asthma, allergies, panic attacks, chronic bronchitis, hay fever, sleeping problems and headaches.

This knowledge was slow to filter through into regular medicine. For many years, former pulmonary function laboratory assistant Stans van der Poel (1955) worked to give breathing and breathing exercises a more prominent place in health care. If you breathe more calmly, your heart rate will slow down and you will improve the ratio of oxygen to carbon dioxide in your blood. Van der Poel developed equipment to measure breathing, respiratory rate, heart rate and heart rate variability. The advantage of this equipment is that you can measure whether specific breathing exercises work or not.

Van der Poel discovered—in addition to Buteyko's diagnoses—that people with chronic fatigue, burnout, fibromyalgia and myalgic encephalomyelitis also breathe more rapidly or deeply than is necessary. Patients who could observe the measurements of their decreased heart rate were motivated to start doing the exercises. Besides the exercises, van der Poel urged people to take up a sport. During fitness activities, breath rate is an important indicator of whether people are overexerting themselves. During a stress test, breathing can also indicate the optimal heart rate for energetic recovery. That is very important to know, especially for people who suffer from fatigue.

Our knowledge of breathing can be used and repurposed in various ways. Because of yoga, meditation, Russian doctors, and a Dutch pulmonary function lab assistant, we now have equipment and a number of apps to help us. Western doctors and ordinary people are now recommending and practicing the exercises, with Wim Hof leading the way.

So why are breathing exercises becoming so popular? To find out, we will first take a look at the physiology of breathing.

OXYGEN AND CARBON DIOXIDE

A quick recap: You breathe oxygen in and carbon dioxide out. Oxygen is transferred to your bloodstream by your lungs and carried around your whole body. Excess carbon dioxide is transported in the opposite direction. The lungs have a hierarchical structure and consist of two parts: the left lung and the right lung.

Oxygen enters the lungs through the windpipe (trachea). It passes through the main bronchus into smaller branches known as bronchioles. The bronchioles come out in the alveoli, the air sacs in the lungs where the oxygen comes into contact with the blood. During this "gas exchange", the ratio of oxygen to carbon dioxide in the lungs and in the blood is the same because of the law of "communicating vessels". The ideal ratio of oxygen to carbon dioxide in the blood is 3:2.

Oxygen is important for releasing energy from nutrients, while carbon dioxide is important for keeping the blood vessels open. Carbon dioxide is often incorrectly seen as waste—something that must be expelled from the body. But, it is essential that your blood vessels stay open so that oxygen can reach everywhere in your body.

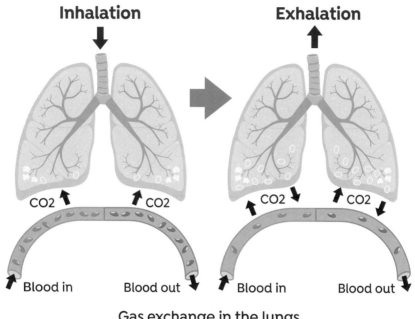

Gas exchange in the lungs

Breathing is not only directly connected to the oxygen and carbon dioxide levels in your blood, but also to your heart rate. Your heart and lungs are inextricably linked to each other. If you breathe faster, your heart rate will almost certainly increase. If you breathe differently, your heart rate changes, as does your heart rate variability. Heart rate variability or heart rate coherence is the variation in time between two successive heartbeats. Someone with a resting heart rate of 60 beats per minute may have a pause of about a second between each beat. But, it is also possible to have intervals between a half and one-and-a-half seconds between beats. The second case is much better than the first.

Contrary to what most people think, it is important for the intervals between heart beats to vary. A healthy heart will beat faster at rest during inhalation than exhalation. In his bestseller, *Healing Without Freud or Prozac*, French psychiatrist David Servan-Schreiber writes extensively on the importance of good heart rate variability. He claims that people suffering from depression, stress, cancer, or who are in the final stages of life have low heart rate variability without exception. Servan-Schreiber backs up these bold claims with a whole series of scientific studies. He also explores the link between heart rate variability and the autonomic nervous system.

In *Healing Without Freud or Prozac*, Servan-Schreiber describes how he no longer helps people with anxiety disorders and depression solely with medication, but also gives them exercises to help improve their heart rate variability. He calls this "complementary treatment". He writes:

"We can witness this interplay between the emotional brain and the heart in the constant variability of the normal heart rate. Because the two branches of the autonomic nervous system are always in equilibrium, they are continually in the process of speeding up and slowing down the heart. That change is why the interval between two successive heartbeats is never identical. This heart rate variability is perfectly healthy; in fact it's a sign of the proper functioning of the brake and the accelerator, and thus of our overall physiological system."

HEART RATE VARIABILITY, THE NERVOUS SYSTEM AND BREATHING

The "brake" and "accelerator" mentioned in the previous quote are also known as the parasympathetic and the sympathetic nervous systems. The sympathetic nervous system is associated with everything to do with action. If it dominates, your body will be in "fight-or-flight" mode. You will breathe faster, your digestive system will stop working momentarily, and your blood will move from your skin to your muscles, internal organs, and your brain. That is why the sympathetic system is often compared to a car's accelerator.

The parasympathetic nervous system regulates everything relating to recovery: a slow heart rate and breathing, a good flow of blood to the skin, and an active digestive system. Therefore, the parasympathetic system is sometimes known as the body's brake pedal.

In their 1989(!) book on the relationship of the parasympathetic nervous system to stress and mental and physical illness, Pieter Langendijk and Agnes van Enkhuizen described the influence of the parasympathetic nervous system on our health. The book also contains concise research data gathered for the Dutch research institute TNO by Professor Tony Gaillard. The results show a direct correlation between decreased activity of the parasympathetic nervous system and physical health problems. It is also clear that breathing exercises can activate your parasympathetic system. (For the record, sex is also primarily a parasympathetic activity).

The graphs on the next page show how breathing influences your heart rate variability.

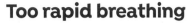

Too rapid breathing

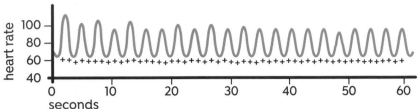

The wavy line is your breathing; it goes up when you breathe in and down when you breathe out. Each time the line goes up then down again is one breathing cycle. The plus signs show heart rate. The vertical axis indicates heartbeats per minute and the horizontal axis is time in seconds. This graph shows the breathing of a 42-year-old woman, sitting on a chair for one minute. Her respiratory rate is 22 and her average heart rate is 61 bpm. Her heart rate is nice and low, but her respiratory rate is high, showing that she is not calm. To further illustrate that, see the graph below which shows her results after practicing breathing exercises for a one minute.

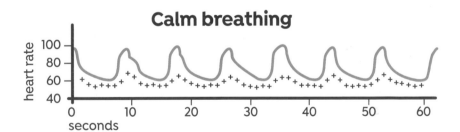

Calm breathing

Her respiratory rate is automatically much lower, since she is now concentrating on her breathing. She now breathes only seven times a minute, rather than twenty-two times. Her respiratory rate falls sharply, and her heart has also responded to the exercise: her average heart rate is a little higher at 62 bpm, but the heart rate variability is noticeably better. As these graphs clearly show, if you have a good breathing pattern, your heart rate varies along with the pattern.

Focused breathing exercises are a very good way to improve your heart rate variability. If you have a clear picture of your heart rate variability, you can determine which breathing exercises work well for you. Stans van der Poel's *Co2ntrol*, for example, can be very effective, but is very expensive for private individuals. You can still do a lot on your own by concentrating on your heart rate. The cheapest heart rate monitors are a good start. Sit down, put on a heart-rate monitor (if you haven't got one, you can probably borrow one from a friend who is a keen sportsman or woman) and check your heart rate after two minutes. Do the breathing exercises described in this chapter and see what happens. If your heart rate varies with your breathing, then everything is OK.

BREATHING AND HEALTH PROBLEMS

Breathing incorrectly can cause a whole range of health problems. We will explain five of them:

1. Pain in the shoulders or neck
2. Agitation
3. Intestinal problems
4. Tiring quickly
5. Heart palpitations

These problems are all related to breathing in different ways.

1. PAIN IN THE SHOULDERS OR NECK

We have accessory respiratory muscles in our necks that help us breathe faster for short periods. If you continually breathe more rapidly than necessary, these muscles will become overtaxed and start to hurt. The pain is similar to the feeling in your leg muscles after running for a long distance. If you rest, the pain in your legs goes away, and the same applies to the muscles in your shoulders or neck. If you breathe more calmly, the pain will disappear.

2. AGITATION

You feel agitated because breathing too quickly will disrupt your body's hormone management. You will produce too much adrenaline and that will make you feel agitated and restless.

3. INTESTINAL PROBLEMS

If the balance between oxygen and carbon dioxide in your blood is disrupted, it will have a strong effect on your intestines. Many people with incorrect breathing patterns feel bloated, belch frequently or suffer from flatulence. These problems can be very inconvenient, even though they are not serious.

4. TIRING QUICKLY

Breathing too fast can make you physically exhausted because you are continually using your high-energy glucose reserves. Roughly speaking, the body has two sources of fuel: fats and glucose. If you breathe too fast, your body uses its glucose reserves more quickly than necessary. We have fewer reserves of glucose than of low-energy fats. Burning up your body's fuel incorrectly in this way means that you will crave sugar and sweet foods more often.

5. HEART PALPITATIONS

Excessive expulsion of carbon dioxide makes your blood vessels contract—the same blood vessels that expand again after exposure to the cold. Your heart tries to compensate for this by pumping blood through your body as quickly as possible. That is a smart response by your body, but it makes a lot of people anxious or short of breath and they often get palpitations.

BREATHING AND SERIOUS STRESS-RELATED DISORDERS

Besides these five common health problems, psychiatrist Bram Bakker also establishes a link between a high respiratory rate and certain psychiatric disorders. The more serious a psychiatric problem is, the more difficult it is to imagine breathing exercises could offer a solution. Yet, it is still worth considering breathing exercises when addressing serious psychiatric disorders.

Breathing too fast is a sign of stress—and, in the case of any stress-related psychological problem, the patient may have a high respiratory rate. Although stress is a factor in most psychological problems, in practice it is primarily and most commonly linked with anxiety disorders and depression. Rapid breathing also plays a significant role in many as yet unexplained physical complaints that affect more and more people.

Stress only appears explicitly in two diagnoses: acute stress disorder and post-traumatic stress disorder. Both disorders can only be diagnosed as such if the patient has had a traumatic experience. This means by definition, unexpected and radical events that could have resulted in serious injury or even death. Such events can lead to stress and psychological problems and can affect the breathing in the short term or more permanently.

Besides these two stress-related disorders, other anxiety disorders are accompanied by agitated breathing. The most common of these is panic disorder, previously known as hyperventilation syndrome. This diagnosis is no longer used since there is no direct causal link between hyperventilation and panic attacks. In other words, hyperventilation does not *always* lead to anxiety attacks, and people suffering from panic attacks do not always hyperventilate. An important point in this discussion is to consider how hyperventilation may be defined. In very clear-cut cases, it makes no difference. For example, what is the significance of a slightly higher respiratory rate in a situation where someone is sitting on the couch at home while breathing twice as rapidly as necessary?

As far as we know, this has not been studied, but we suspect that many people who suffer from an anxiety disorder have an excessively high respiratory rate at rest.

Breathing and relaxation exercises have been widely researched and have been found to be effective for anxiety disorders. Yet, they are hardly used by psychologists and psychiatrists. "Applied relaxation" is in the official guidelines for treating general anxiety disorder, but only if cognitive therapy is not available or cannot be applied for some reason. Cognitive therapy only works for people of average or higher intelligence, while applied relaxation—like the WHM—works for everyone. Applied relaxation can be used to help someone recognize the early signals of panic and gain control through relaxation exercises. First, the patient will learn to relax. Then, relaxation can be associated with a certain word that has a calming effect. When panic signals occur, this word can be used to stop the panic from getting worse.

Our short detour into psychiatry was to emphasize the importance of breathing for treating a wide range of health problems—and to show that there are other exercises besides the WHM breathing exercises that can be used for relaxation.

WHY DO MANY PEOPLE BREATHE SO RAPIDLY?

Why do so many of us breathe incorrectly? Breathing calmly should be as automatic as many of our other bodily functions. Our body temperature is always 36.8°C (98.2°F), our hearts keep on beating, and our eyes blink by themselves. Why don't we breathe calmly as a matter of course—especially if it is healthier for us? It seems that excessive stimulation, worry, preoccupation, and persistent mental pressure all affect our breathing.

Breathing and the Brain

The neocortex is the part of the brain that distinguishes humans from other animals. "Neo" means "new" in Latin and, in evolutionary terms, the neocortex is the youngest part of the brain. We use it to analyze and calculate, and it is also our language center. But, it is also the part of the brain that allows us to worry about what will happen in two weeks' time—or allows us to stay irritated about a past event.

The "mammalian" or emotional brain is where we process the emotions we share with other mammals, such as fear, aggression, love and sorrow. The limbic system is found in this part of the brain.

A layer deeper is the reptilian brain, where we find the functions we share with reptiles. Our blood pressure, heart rate, and breathing are regulated here. Likewise, the reptilian brain keeps our body temperature at 36.8°C, without our conscious attention.

The neocortex also filters external stimuli. Research has shown that today we are exposed to as many external stimuli in one day as someone living in the Middle Ages encountered during a lifetime. We make an average of 2,800 choices each day—every day. So, it is not surprising that at some point, we will receive too many signals to handle. One way the resulting agitation manifests itself is in more rapid breathing.

An over-stimulated neocortex can make us breathe faster. But you can also use the neocortex to slow down your breathing.

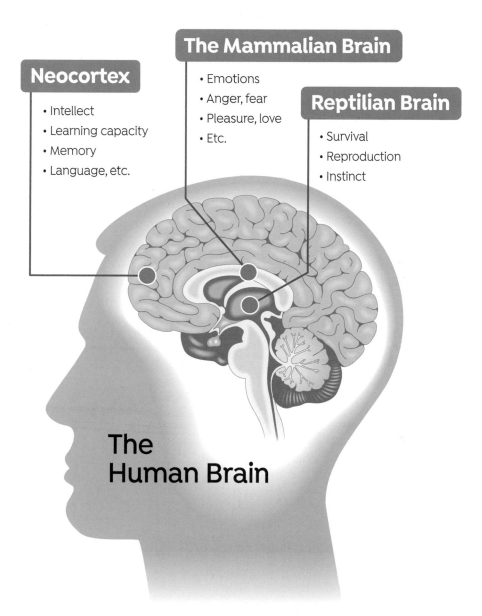

Neocortex
- Intellect
- Learning capacity
- Memory
- Language, etc.

The Mammalian Brain
- Emotions
- Anger, fear
- Pleasure, love
- Etc.

Reptilian Brain
- Survival
- Reproduction
- Instinct

The
Human Brain

BREATHING EXERCISES TO HELP YOU RELAX

The exercises in my book, *Verademing*, are mainly focused on relaxation, and restoring a normal balance between oxygen and carbon dioxide in the body.

Here are two breathing exercises that are good for relaxation:

- Breathe in through your nose
- Breathe out through your nose
- Pause

- Breathe in through your nose
- Breathe out through your nose
- Pause

Don't pause as long as possible, but just until you feel the need to breathe in again.

If this exercise doesn't relax you, breathe out through your mouth:

- Breathe in through your nose
- Breathe out through your mouth, prolonging the breath a little
- Pause

- Breathe in through your nose
- Breathe out through your mouth, prolonging the breath a little
- Pause

You can easily prolong your breath by holding back so that your cheeks puff out a little as you breathe out. It is good to relax by practicing these breathing exercises for two minutes before you start doing the WHM exercises. The WHM exercises are completely different and serve a different purpose—which will be explained later.

THE WHM BREATHING EXERCISES

The Wim Hof breathing exercises are not intended to relax you—at least not while you are doing them. They are designed to enable you to control your mind and body, so you can influence your autonomic nervous system.

At first, the WHM exercises will make you light-headed. It is hard work to keep your attention focused while doing the exercises properly.

So far, we have only referred to breathing exercises and not to meditation. Yet, Hof's exercises have their origins in a Tibetan technique known as Tummo meditation.

Tummo is a form of meditation with its roots in the Indian Vajrayana tradition. Vajrayana is a religion that probably emerged around the fourth century AD, and which was heavily influenced by Tantric and Hindu teaching. Vajrayana works from a cause and effect perspective. The aim is to transform every experience into fearless wisdom, spontaneous joy and energetic love. Hof emphasizes that this does not necessitate or imply faith in a higher power—rather, that what you experience be true for yourself. Followers of Vajrayana see the method as the most important link in achieving enlightenment through the Buddha's teaching.

TUMMO TECHNIQUE

Tummo combines breathing with visualization. It involves breathing in deeply and breathing out slowly. While breathing, practitioners visualize flames, as a method to help raise their body temperature. Because they focus on experience and not on faith, they also embrace science. In the scientific journal *PLOS ONE*, researchers from the National University of Singapore described their study of nuns who practiced Tummo meditation. They discovered that the nuns could generate extra body heat, increasing their temperatures to 38.3°C (100.9°F), in an ambient temperature of -25°C (-13°F). With their bodies, they were also able to dry wet clothes which were wrapped around them.

Wim Hof did not study Tummo directly. He learned everything from nature, not from a religion. However, after his own experience, a knowledge of Tummo helped Wim gain a deeper understanding of the power of cold. And what most appeals to him is the idea that Vajrayana is a religion based on experience, not faith. It is about experiencing, not believing. Every proposition can ultimately be checked against your own experience. One of Wim's favorite one-liners is: "feeling is understanding". And that's exactly what the Tummo techniques encourage.

DO-IT-YOURSELF:
THE WHM BREATHING EXERCISES

A word of warning in advance: Don't do this breathing exercise in a position or location where fainting might be dangerous, such as in the shower, underwater, while standing up, or in the car. Do it under supervision the first time.

- Breathe in deeply, and then exhale
- Breathe in deeply, and then exhale
- Breathe in deeply, and then exhale

— Breathe at a pace and rhythm that feel most comfortable
— Repeat this 30 times
— The last time, breathe out completely, then in again very deeply, out again slowly, and then wait.

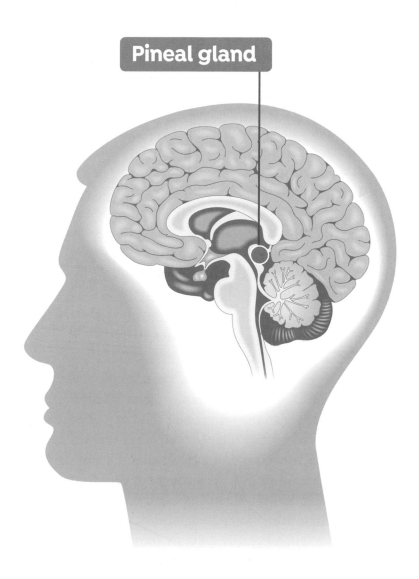

Pineal gland

Breathe in deeply, without forcing yourself, and then out again slowly. By not fully breathing out, a small amount of air remains behind in the lungs. After doing that 30 times, hold your breath after breathing out, and wait until you feel the need to breathe in again. Repeat this exercise until you feel tingling, light in the head, or sluggish.

By breathing in deeply and out slowly, you expel a lot of carbon dioxide. The CO_2 concentration in your blood will decrease and your blood vessels will contract. When you hold your breath after breathing out, your body retains a large quantity of carbon dioxide, and your body compensates by releasing more oxygen in the mitochondria. Mitochondria supply the energy for your body's cells. More oxygen in the mitochondria generates more energy. Waste substances are expelled and the oxygen has more room to penetrate deeper into the cell. Holding your breath after exhaling leads to a parasympathetic reaction (in other words, you relax). This leads to aerobic dissimilation in the cell. By breathing more deeply and consciously, we can therefore generate more energy in the cell.

PINEAL GLAND

After these breathing exercises, many people experience an expanded form of consciousness. This is likely from the mitochondrial activity in the brain cells releasing chemicals in the pituitary and pineal glands. The pineal gland (epiphysis cerebri) is very important for determining our state of mind. It produces melatonin, a hormone that plays an important role in our sleep-wake and reproductive rhythms. Our hypothesis is—that through the WHM breathing exercises—much more oxygen enters the pineal gland, so the body will generate a lot more oxygen. That explains why the exercises work so well in combating jetlag, sleeping problems and depression.

Interestingly, in Eastern philosophies, the pineal gland is seen as the seat of the soul. The French philosopher René Descartes (1596-1650) also considered it to be the link between body and soul. He was one of the first Western thinkers to "promote" the pineal gland.

BREATH RETENTION

You can check whether your body changes during the breathing exercises by measuring how long you can hold your breath. Check how long you can hold your breath before doing the exercises, and then again afterwards. You will notice that you can hold your breath longer and longer.

It is good if your retention time (the time between breathing out and back in again) gets longer, but don't make a competition out of it. It is a way to determine if the method is working, not an end in itself.

SUMMARY

- Many people breathe quicker or deeper than necessary
- A disrupted breathing pattern is related to a series of health problems
- Breathing exercises affect brain activity
- There are exercises you can use to relax
- The WHM uses breathing to access the pineal gland
- Oxygen activates the expulsion of waste substances
- Carbon dioxide opens the blood vessels

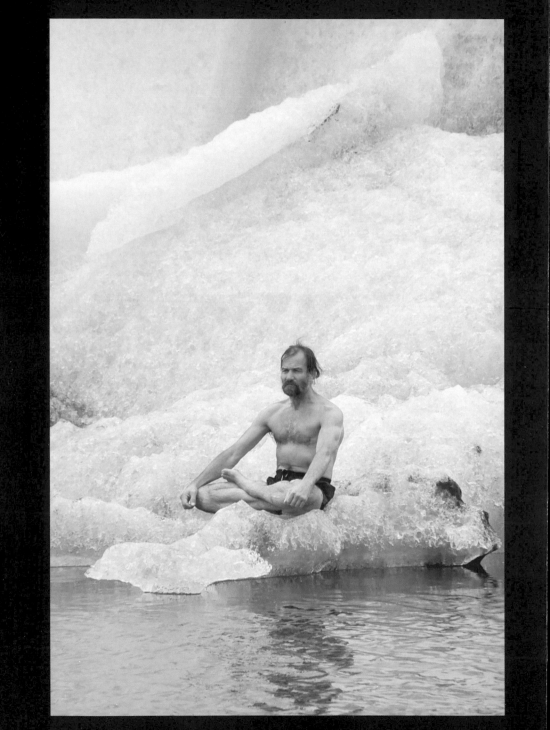

COMMITMENT

The cold training and breathing exercises are two major components of the Wim Hof Method. But to properly put these two components into practice, you need to make a serious commitment.

Especially at first, it is not easy to turn off the warm water and stand under a cold shower for two minutes. Those two minutes seem to last forever. And daily breathing exercises are quite a task, too. Where will you find the time? And the motivation?

A day with Wim Hof will give you motivation enough. His enthusiasm and experience will encourage you to get started with his method. This has nothing to do with behavior-changing approaches like neuro-linguistic programming (NLP). It is simply an overwhelming enthusiasm that seems to come from the depths of his soul.

To help motivate you to take cold showers and give the breathing exercises a try, we will describe a fantastic example of what your body is capable of if you make a serious commitment.

Running a Marathon
Bare-Chested Above the Arctic Circle

Wim Hof underwent an extreme challenge to demonstrate how making a commitment and controlling your mind are more important than physical training. He ran a marathon above the Arctic Circle. This was the most difficult test he had ever undertaken.

Hof took on this challenge in 2009, at the age of 50. Running a marathon at -16°C (3.2°F) was not enough, he ran only wearing shorts and sandals with no socks. He did this to test his knowledge of his body. He knew that a lot is possible, but he didn't just want to pass that knowledge to others at an intellectual level—Wim wanted to experience it himself.

His preparation training and the marathon in Finland were filmed by Firecrackerfilms, a company that frequently works for the BBC and National Geographic. The documentary was later shown on the television program, *Daredevils*.

Physical Training—
or Training the Commitment?

People who prepare for marathons in normal temperatures usually have training programs and gradually build up their running distances. But, Wim didn't use a training program and hardly went running at all. He just trained with the cold and his thoughts, while focusing on the commitment.

Hof prepared by doing extra breathing exercises and cold training. In the winter, he swam in the canals in Amsterdam at night. To get accustomed to even more extreme conditions, he trained in the cold storage at a slaughterhouse where the temperature was -25°C (-13°F). He practiced his breathing techniques and grew increasingly confident that he could take on the challenge. After the training sessions, he felt strong and in good spirits.

Glyn David, an expert on polar survival, had serious misgivings. Breathing is extremely difficult at such temperatures and running makes you breathe more deeply. He felt that it was practically impossible to do that for hours on end in such conditions.

In Finland

Hof went to Finland six days before the marathon. It was cold, even by Finnish standards. The day before the marathon, he practiced once more in the extreme cold by swimming for several dozen meters under the ice. Doctors who examined him on the spot couldn't understand it—his heart rate, blood pressure and oxygen saturation were the same before and after he had been swimming. Hof felt good and decided he was ready for the challenge.

During the marathon, Hof was constantly balancing on a fine thread. If he ran too fast, he used too much energy and had to breathe in too deeply—which is not possible at 16°C below zero (3.2°F). If he ran too slowly, he would be exposed to the cold for too long and would risk suffering the serious effects of freezing.

After running for two hours, everything was still going fine. His legs felt heavy, but his pace was still constant. At that point, he had run about half of the 42,195 meters (26.2 miles). However, at 30 kilometers (18.6 miles), and running for a little over three hours, fatigue set in. He was clearly tired and suffering from the cold. His second wife, Caroline, was ahead of him in a car with the film crew and a doctor. She was worried because the situation could become very dangerous. But Hof kept going, even when he had to walk after 37 kilometers (23 miles). After 5 hours and 25 minutes, Hof had accomplished the impossible: he ran a marathon above the Arctic Circle in extremely cold temperatures—bare-chested—with no marathon training.

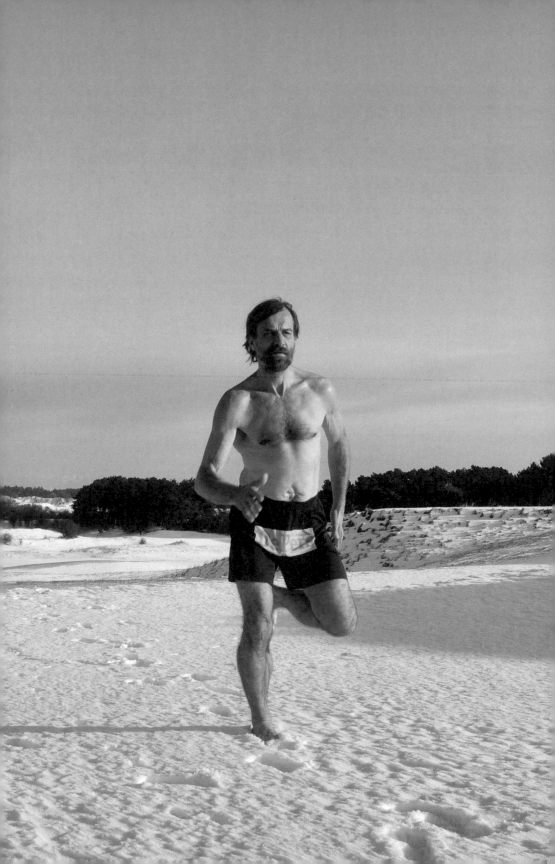

Such an extreme commitment only seems possible for exceptional individuals like Wim Hof. But he refuses to believe that and to prove it years later, he decided to go to the top of Mount Kilimanjaro with a group of people—to do the impossible as a group.

MOUNT KILIMANJARO

Hof decided he would climb Mount Kilimanjaro with a group of people. Kilimanjaro is a 5,895 meter (3.66 mile) high mountain in Tanzania. It's a very popular expedition for mountaineers and hikers. Well-trained climbers can get to the top in six days.

To make the challenge even greater, Hof wanted to climb Kilimanjaro in 48 hours with a group of 26 people. Hof wanted to show that we are all capable of doing much more than most people think is even possible. With this expedition, too, everyone said it was impossible to get to the top in 48 hours with such a large group.

As if that wasn't enough, some of the people in the group were suffering from diseases like multiple sclerosis, rheumatism, Crohn's disease and cancer. They also had no climbing experience.

The date was set for January 2014, and the run up to the expedition was chaotic. Dr. Geert Buijze of the Amsterdam Medical Centre wanted to accompany the expedition in a personal capacity to help the group. The local guides thought the whole thing was a bad idea. At the last moment, the guides decided not to go. However, Hof was resolute that this group was capable of reaching the top by focusing on their breathing and because they had prepared with cold training. So, they went.

When the group arrived at Horombo Hut—a small huddle of climbing huts at an altitude of 3,705 meters (2.3 miles)—the temperature had fallen to 3°C (37.4°F). As if climbing to the top of

Kilimanjaro in 48 hours with 26 people, many of whom were ill, was not enough, Wim suggested they walk bare-chested and in shorts. Breathing and cold training were the secrets.

He gave instructions to his mixed bunch of companions, then divided them into pairs. Each partner had to watch out for each other—and in particular, they had to make sure to keep doing their breathing exercises. They had to keep breathing in deeply, and exhaling calmly and slowly. To combat altitude sickness, they also woke up during the night to keep performing the breathing exercises.

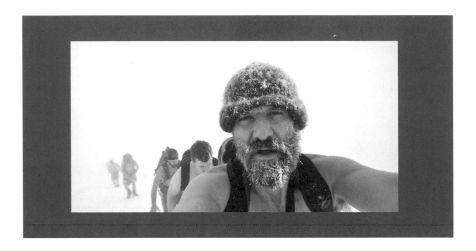

To everyone's amazement—except Hof's of course—the group performed an exceptional feat. Twenty-four of the 26 reached Uhuru Peak, the top of the mountain at 5,895 meters (3.66 miles). The temperature at the peak was -15°C (5°F). The fact that such a large group had reached the top was an achievement in itself. It was extra special since the group had no climbing experience. When they reached the top within 48 hours, it was almost impossible to comprehend. The feat attracted the attention of the media. Hof and Buijze found themselves sitting at the table on *Pauw en Witteman*, a leading Dutch current affairs program. Several newspapers carried stories about the triumph.

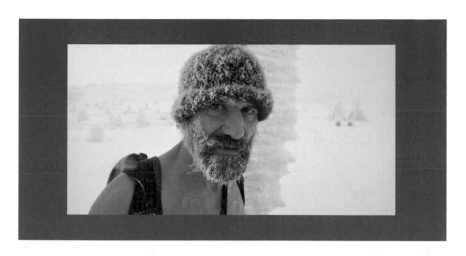

How was something like this possible?

Hof is convinced of the power of his breathing exercises. And although the group had no climbing experience, they were well trained to withstand the cold. Commitment to the feat was of course an important factor.

The members of the group who were suffering with diseases included Anna Chojnacka (MS), Mark Bos (prostate cancer), Henk van den Bergh (rheumatism) and Mathijs Storm and Hans Emmink (Crohn's disease). They all walked to the summit, too.

All of these people knew they were ill, but they did not see themselves as patients. They made that clear time and again. This idea proves to be an important component of the commitment. "Of course I'm a patient, too," says Mathijs Storm, "but I'm also just Mathijs who wants to—and can—do all kinds of things."

KILIMANJARO 2015

In January 2015, Hof returned to Kilimanjaro with a new group. This time, the goal was to get to the top in 36 hours. Once again, Hof wanted to show people that they can accomplish much more than they might imagine. The WHM exercises worked well—15 of the 19 participants succeeded in completing the climb bare-chested.

The group did not climb all the way to Uhuru Peak, but stopped at Gilman's Point, on the rim of the crater at 5,685 meters (3.53 miles). The group chose safety over their egos. One of the members proposed to his wife at Gilman's Point.

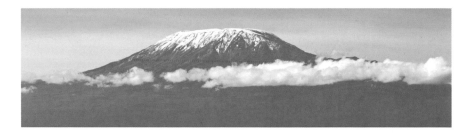

SIDE EFFECTS OF THE WHM

The Wim Hof Method comprises three components: cold training, breathing exercises and commitment. It also involves more. The interviews conducted for this book showed that people who did cold training and breathing exercises, found that other things in their lives changed too.

They slept better, walked or played a sport more often, and appreciated the daylight more. We are not going to examine all these changes, but two were particularly noticeable, as they were often mentioned: walking barefoot and eating less.

WALKING BAREFOOT

A surprising number of people who use the WHM start walking barefoot. After ten interviews, eight of the interviewees had started walking barefoot—it can't be a coincidence. Hof himself doesn't pay much attention to it, but he often walks barefoot, too.

Many people consider walking barefoot to be healthy. Once you start looking for it, you see how many people run barefoot, and the subject crops up regularly in newspapers and magazines. The main message of these articles is that walking barefoot strengthens the muscles in the foot—muscles that are hardly used when you wear shoes—and increases your bone mass. The feet contain 200,000 nerve endings which sounds like an enormous amount. It explains why walking barefoot is so sensitive. Setting your feet down lightly can feel very pleasant and comfortable; to some people, it feels like a massage. We also walk differently on our bare feet, and put more weight on the front of our feet.

Steven Robbins and Adel Hanna's study of 17 recreational runners in 1987 showed that after four months of not wearing shoes, the longitudinal arch of the foot was shortened by an average of 4.7 millimeters (3/16"). Robbins and Hanna suggested that this change must have been caused by the enhanced activation of the foot muscles, and that this may help in reducing or preventing stress on the plantar fascia, on the underside of the foot. This worked well in the study, because the transition to running barefoot was gradual. Studies where the change happened too quickly reported an increased risk of foot injury.

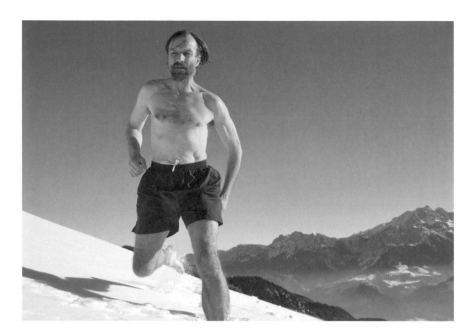

EARTHING

Proponents of walking barefoot emphasize that "earthing"—making contact with the Earth's electrical field—has a favorable effect on health. The Earth is negatively charged while the air is full of positive ions. The quantity of positive ions has greatly increased in recent years with the widespread use of radios, televisions, cell phones, and other forms of wireless communications. Too many positive ions can disrupt the balance between positive and negative.

"Because of our modern lifestyles, we have become isolated from the Earth—not a healthy situation," says electrical engineer, Clinton Ober. He discovered the positive health effects of earthing, which connects us with the negative electrons on the Earth's surface.

Can you counteract the surplus of positive electrons by being in contact with the Earth? That's a tough question. The contact is partly thwarted by thick rubber soles, which insulate us from the electrical discharge. Walking barefoot puts you in direct contact with the earth, and that gives you more energy.

One interviewee who said that he now walks barefoot more often is Richard de Leth. De Leth studied medicine at the VU University in Amsterdam and applies a mix of Western and Eastern medicine in his practice. His book *Oersterk*, which has sold more than 70,000 copies, is an appeal to people to eat healthier foods. One of his pet topics is eating less sugar. De Leth has a favorite quote, by T.S. Eliot, who won the Nobel Prize for Literature in 1948:

"Where is the wisdom we have lost in knowledge?
Where is the knowledge we have lost in information?"

In his quest for wisdom, De Leth came across Wim Hof. In 2013, he took part in one of Hof's workshops. He did the breathing exercises and sat in a bath of ice cubes. He described his experiences that day as exceptional. After only a few exercises, he could hold his breath for 2.5 minutes and did 60 push-ups without breathing. The ice bath felt good, too. His body turned red immediately, a sign of good circulation.

Several months after the workshop, we asked De Leth whether he still uses the methods he learned. He said he still does the breathing exercises and looks forward to the snow in winter so that he can go barefoot outside. What has changed permanently for him is walking barefoot much more often, in the house and outside—and that it feels good.

Diet

Many people who start applying the Wim Hof Method also start eating differently. Hof hardly eats at all—he rarely has breakfast and doesn't eat lunch. He only eats in the evenings, but as much as he wants and whatever he feels like eating. Jack Egberts was one of the first people to study Hof's eating habits. Jack is the lawyer from Leeuwaarden who we mentioned earlier in the chapter about cold training. We will examine his detective work more closely here, because his results show parallels with the WHM. Jack's approach to eating is simple to do, but effectively penetrates to the core of many diseases related to prosperity.

Egberts discovered a dietary philosophy very similar to the way Hof eats, the "fast-5 diet". Just to be clear, Wim does not encourage people to actively adopt this way of eating, but eats this way instinctively. What Hof and Jack Egberts do can be summed up very simply:

Eat during a five-hour period each day, no more.

The fast-5 diet was (re)discovered by Bert Herring, a former Air Force doctor. As a doctor, he knew that there is no physiological reason for all men and women over the age of 40 to become overweight. And yet, in the mirror he saw a man with a large double chin, breasts, and a belly. He wanted to get rid of his excess weight. But, instead of going straight to the gym, he first went to the library. He learned more about diseases of prosperity and their causes. He re-read his old textbooks. He discovered that it is not only important what we eat, but how often.

Often, other large mammals eat only once a day. They are hardly ever overweight and rarely suffer from cardiovascular disease, diabetes or cancer. Since we are also large mammals, Herring felt that people are not made to eat all day. He talked to his wife Judi— also a doctor and a few pounds too heavy—about it, and they decided to do an experiment together.

For a month, they ate as much as they liked and whatever they liked, but only between five in the afternoon and ten o'clock at night. The results were astounding. Herring saw muscles appearing in places where he only knew of their existence because of his anatomical knowledge. He shed the pounds, his blood pressure fell, his gums were no longer infected. He felt much more energetic and had the desire to go running. The same thing happened to his wife. She was also pleasantly surprised at the effects. Curious friends adopted the new eating habits and experienced similar results.

Herring decided to name the method of eating for only five hours a day the "fast-5 diet". He wrote an e-book about it, which he made available for free on the internet. The former Air Force doctor said that he didn't want to earn money from such a simple physiological truth. He emphasized that the basis of his method could be written on the back of a beer-mat: only eat for a period of five hours a day. In the book, he explains that this practice trains your body to mainly use fat as fuel instead of glucose. This idea also ties in with the production of brown fat during cold training.

At first, like Jack Egberts, most people will still feel hungry. At five o'clock in the afternoon, they will likely have a serious attack of "the munchies". That is normal. But after a few days, that desire will have almost disappeared. There's no need to fight against it, as the desire will soon weaken. You don't need to worry about fainting— even though you might feel a bit weak in the first few days—unless you have diabetes and don't adapt your medication.

The "fast-5 diet" way of eating imposes no restrictions on your calorie intake, but soon you start to automatically eat less. That is why it is important to mainly eat food with a high nutritional value. Herring recommends a combination of vegetables, fruit, meat, fish and chicken to provide a good variety. You will notice as your body becomes accustomed to this "simpler" diet, and as you use up more fat than glucose, you will lose around 300 grams (0.66 pounds) a week. Your energy levels will also be more constant.

Now that we have described the Wim Hof Method and the link between breathing, cold and commitment, what does science say about the WHM? In the next chapter, we describe the research conducted at the Radboud Medical Centre and the remarkable insights of Professor Pierre Capel.

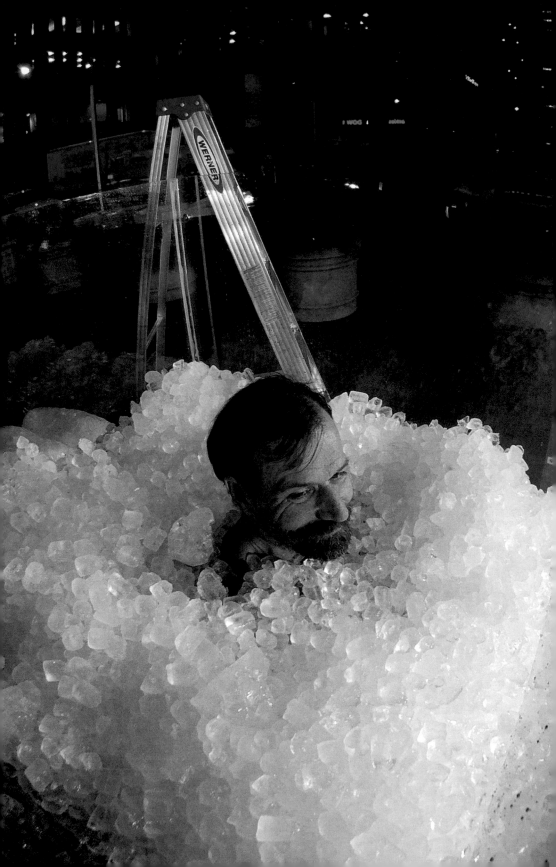

Science

"I am a scientist: my body is my laboratory."
–Wim Hof

With his extreme feats, Wim Hof has also attracted the attention of scientists. Researchers are queuing up to explain his exceptional achievements. What Hof does with his body defies everything that can be found in medical textbooks.

In 2011, the Radboud University Medical Centre in Nijmegen started a long-term study of Hof and his method.

First, they studied Hof as an individual. Hof claims that he can influence his autonomic nervous system and his immune system. It is extraordinary—it goes against everything doctors learn when they are studying medicine.

What is the Autonomic Nervous System?

We discussed the autonomic nervous system earlier in the chapter on breathing. Just to recap: your body is active every second of your life, without your conscious thought. Your intestines are active, your pupils dilate or constrict, your heart beats, your body remains at a constant temperature and billions of cells are constantly in motion. All these bodily functions work automatically.

Hence the name, autonomic nervous system—it works on its own, without your control. The nervous system has two components: the parasympathetic and the sympathetic systems. In simple terms, the parasympathetic system is the brake and the sympathetic system is the gas pedal.

Another system we are told we cannot influence is our natural immune system, which also works without our conscious awareness. The natural immune system is a very old evolutionary defense system that combats viruses, bacteria and other external threats to our bodies.

Medical science reports that we cannot consciously influence either our autonomic nervous system or our natural immune system.

Wim Hof disagrees.

To investigate whether Hof really is capable of influencing his natural immune system, the researchers injected him with endotoxin, a strong toxin found in the cell walls of certain bacteria. Our natural immune system has been programmed for hundreds of millions of years to respond immediately to this toxin. Special receptors on white corpuscles, known as Toll-like receptors (TLR), bind to the endotoxin and produce inflammatory proteins. This can be compared to a reflex reaction and cannot be controlled.

Besides Hof, a control group of twelve people were also given an endotoxin injection. As a result of the response from their immune systems, the test subjects developed flu-like symptoms, including fever, shivering and headaches. But, Hof did his breathing exercises and to the researchers' amazement developed no symptoms at all. His body was clearly able to deal with the endotoxin. During this experiment, the researchers found indications in Hof's blood of heightened activity in the sympathetic nervous system. His adrenaline level went up even before the endotoxin was injected. Far fewer inflammatory proteins were found, while the initial increase in his cortisol level decreased much more quickly than among the control group.

This experiment suggested that the prevailing belief in medical science that we cannot influence our autonomic nervous or natural immune systems was no longer valid. At least, in Wim Hof's case.

"I had to go very deep in this experiment. My body was exposed to a dose of toxin and I had to fight it. But that wasn't the most difficult part. For many years, I've been seen as a fairground attraction, and I was the butt of scorn and cynicism. But I knew that I could influence my autonomous nervous system, and it was tough waiting for recognition. I'm over the moon that Professor Pickkers has now proved scientifically that I really can do it."

—Wim Hof

What does this mean for people with autoimmune diseases? Can they use Hof's method to combat their illness? The researchers were not prepared to make that claim—yet. Although Hof was monitored intensively with all kinds of medical instruments during this experiment and his blood was tested, there was no hard scientific evidence. One finding in the case of one individual proves nothing.

So, in 2013, the researchers decided to conduct a follow-up test. The experiment was repeated with 24 young, healthy male volunteers, randomly selected from many more who applied to take part in the test. The volunteers were then divided into two groups. 12 learned Wim's method in a week, and the other 12 did not. All of the test subjects were then given an endotoxin injection. The 12 men who hadn't learned the WHM showed varying responses. Some hardly had any reaction, but the majority developed a fever. The twelve who learned the method all stayed healthy.

Peter Pickkers, professor of Experimental Intensive Care Medicine at Radboud UMC, led the research team. His research group has been studying infections, immune systems, and how we can influence them for many years.

"That an individual can actively and consciously control his immune system is unique."

—Professor Peter Pickkers

At first, Pickkers remained extremely cautious. The fact that we could influence our immune systems does not necessarily mean that people with chronic illnesses might be able to benefit from the information.

The laboratory measurements were crucial for the definitive results of the test. The fact that the 12 men trained in the WHM did not respond to the endotoxin injection was only a small part of the research.

SCIENTIFIC BREAKTHROUGH

The laboratory results confirmed that after a brief training on how to use the WHM, the 12 men could influence their autonomic nervous systems. For the first time, this had been scientifically illustrated.

The researchers were really enthusiastic about the differences in immune response between the two groups. Pickkers had been skeptical at the start of the research, but now resolutely believed that people are able to influence their autonomic nervous systems.

Immediately after they started applying his method, the men trained in the Wim Hof Method had increased adrenaline levels. In addition, the anti-inflammatory protein IL-10 also increased, repressing the inflammatory proteins IL-6, IL-8 and TNF-α. The control group's adrenaline levels remained low along with their levels of anti-inflammatory proteins. Consequently their inflammatory proteins stayed high.

The men in the trained group showed that they could consciously influence their autonomic nervous systems and their natural immune systems' reaction to endotoxin.

Now, the question was if the method was applicable for people suffering from inflammatory diseases. Pickkers was still extremely cautious on that score. He did indicate that the adrenaline values of the trained men were very promising. It was very significant that this group could drive their adrenaline up higher than someone doing a bungee jump. Adrenaline is very important because we know that adrenaline represses the inflammatory process. Chronic stress is unhealthy, but controlled and acute stress is one of our body's own medicines.

Many medicines have the sole purpose of repressing the inflammation mechanism. All of the anti-inflammatory medicines—such as the best-known example, prednisone–have the disadvantage of extensive and severe side-effects. Adrenaline produced by our own bodies is a natural and healthier alternative. Pickkers adds that we are happy if pharmaceuticals are 20% effective. The WHM-trained group achieved 50% effectiveness using their bodies' own adrenaline.

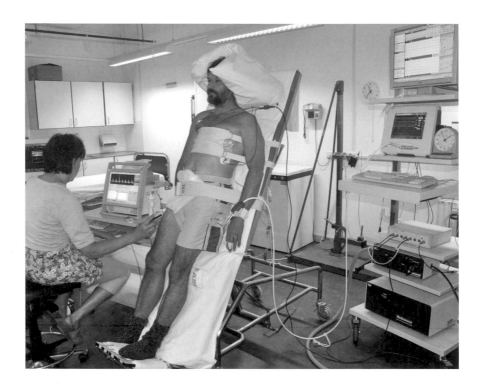

TIP OF THE ICEBERG

The results of the research were published in leading journals like *Nature* and *PNAS*. After the publication, Wim expected an eruption of enthusiasm because the possibilities of his method had been scientifically confirmed. But to his amazement and disappointment, the revelations received little attention. Opinionmakers and the public at large did not immediately see the potential. Interestingly, the results of the research were announced a day before the wildly popular Eurovision Song Festival.

Still, the value of the research had genuinely been recognized.

Immediately after the results were published, Professor of Clinical Chemistry Frits Muskiet said on national Dutch radio that they had "put their fingers on practically all diseases of prosperity".

"Our bodies," Muskiet explained, "continually combat and destroy infections. It should be in balance, but it isn't. Because of our current lifestyles, we live with permanent low levels of infection. You could say that we are chronically infected, but because it is so low, we don't feel it at all. We don't notice it, but it is the breeding ground of many diseases. The experimental group has shown us that it is possible to repress that inflammatory response. I hope that this leads to much more research."

Professor Pierre Capel is a biochemist and immunologist. He goes a step further and feels that meditation, breathing techniques and cold training offer many more possibilities. In his view, Pickkers' explanation is only the tip of the iceberg.

What Do We Know at This Point?

The most important thing we know for certain is that Wim Hof's method works not only for him, but also for other people. That finding excludes the possibility that his results were obtained from a rare combination of biological characteristics. We now know the WHM is broadly applicable. Breathing exercises, meditation and cold training bring about genuine changes in the very important systems of our bodies that we thought until now were beyond our influence. As a result, our immune reactions change and we are capable of greater physical feats—like Hof and his group climbing Mount Kilimanjaro in record time.

What Biological Mechanisms Underlie These Changes?

Let's start with the most difficult component: ice-cold water. To understand how cold water training works, we need to learn how temperature receptors respond, and what they do to our bodies. The family of receptors known as "transient receptor potential (TRP) channels" respond to a variety of stimuli—including temperature changes—and trigger a wide range of processes in the body. There are even special TRP channels for individual temperature ranges. These ranges include heat higher than 42°C (107.7°F), for warmth between 22°C and 41°C (71.6° F-105.8°F), for cold below 22°C (71.6 °F), and severe cold below 7°C (44.6°F). In the presence of heat or cold, the TRPs are linked to pain receptors. When you sit in an ice bath, you will feel cold and pain. Your natural reflex is to get out immediately.

HOW DO PAIN RECEPTORS WORK AND WHAT IS PAIN?

If you tap your finger, you will feel the contact but no pain. But if your finger is inflamed, tapping it can be extremely painful. The inflamed finger does not have more pain receptors, but the receptors it has are more sensitive.

And now it gets a little complicated.

How do receptors become more or less sensitive? A receptor consists of a protein called ASIC, and if three of these proteins form a single complex, they can trigger a pain stimulus.

Pain stimulus also depends on the degree of acidity (pH value) of the body. When the pH value is normal (7.4), only a small percentage of pain receptors are active. If the pH falls, the pain increases, but if it rises, the pain nearly disappears. Besides pain, these receptors also trigger fear and a severe stress response. So if you immerse yourself in ice water unprepared, you will feel pain, fear, panic and severe stress.

So, why doesn't Wim Hof experience this intense reaction? How he can stay in ice-cold water for a long time without his body temperature cooling to any significant degree?

What is the secret?

That's where the breathing comes in. Through Hof's special breathing technique, his pH rises as high as 7.7, and his pain receptors become inactive. If you get into cold water after doing this breathing exercise, you won't feel any pain, panic, or stress because the pain center in the brain is not activated.

The temperature receptors still work, but they are no longer linked to pain or fear. The cold receptors send a signal to the body to burn brown fat, quickly releasing a large amount of calories. The circulation in the epidermis (the outer layer of the skin) is also closed off, so that the body loses less heat. Together, these functions ensure that body temperature hardly falls, allowing Hof to swim in the cold water without suffering hypothermia. But this is not the whole story.

Capel's study showed that the breathing exercises, meditation and cold training have an enormous impact on our DNA. The biochemist explains that every cell in our bodies contains the same DNA—essentially all the required information for every bodily function. Your heart, liver, hands, and teeth all have the same DNA. Yet, no hair grows on your teeth and your heart works in a completely different way than your liver. For example, in the cells of your heart, some of the functions in the DNA are "switched off", while others are "on". Switching genes on and off is an important process. It is regulated by "transcription factors".

A transcription factor is a kind of DNA switch. For every gene, there is a DNA code recognized by a specific transcription factor. When the factor binds to this code, it initiates a complex process, which transforms the information contained in the gene into a protein with a specific function. One transcription factor regulates hundreds of different genes. If just one factor is active or inactive, there is a great impact on hundreds of different functions in our bodies.

Besides the specific genes that always remain "on" or "off" (so that a liver cell is a liver cell and not a kidney cell), there are also genes that are switched on and off in response to external circumstances, such as social contact, eating, or exercising. So engaging happily in sports or other physical activities sends different signals to our genes than does slouching grumpily on the couch.

Of the hundreds of transcription factors, only one is of special interest to us: the nuclear factor kappa b, NF-kB for short. This factor underlies many very important biological processes, including how our immune systems function and how cancer develops. It is widely known that inflammation processes lie at the root of many diseases. NF-kB is a recurring determinant factor in chronic and exhausting inflammatory reactions.

How Does This Relate to Wim Hof and His Method?

Pickkers discovered that Hof can regulate several of his own inflammatory proteins, including IL-6, IL-8 and TNF-α. According to Capel, these proteins are controlled by NF-kB. Through meditation, breathing exercises, and cold training, Hof can influence his NF-kB activity. But, it is not that simple—we must look further than just NF-kB. The world of transcription factors is tangled with many factors working with and against each other.

Another important player in this complex system is CREB. CREB can inhibit NF-kB. In very many processes, CREB and NF-kB are activated simultaneously, usually with the NF-kB response dominant. The response to endotoxin is one process where NF-kB has the upper hand. Under the control of NF-kB, the level of inflammatory proteins goes up, resulting in fever and other symptoms of sickness.

But, when Wim and his trained group were injected with endotoxin, a completely opposite reaction occurred. Their adrenaline levels rose immediately when they started their special breathing exercises. This activated CREB and made it dominant so the inflammatory proteins controlled by NF-kB remained at a low level, while proteins like IL-10—regulated by CREB—increased. As IL-10 also inhibits the inflammatory reaction, the inflammation was doubly inhibited.

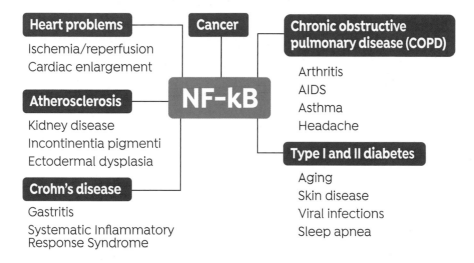

There are many links between NF-kB and diseases of prosperity

WHY IS IT SO IMPORTANT FOR TRANSCRIPTION FACTORS TO BE BALANCED?

As the figure above shows, a large number of diseases are directly related to NF-kB activity.

Chronic stress drives up very high levels of NF-kB activity. If you can influence your NF-kB, you can have an enormously favorable impact on your health. Instead of stress affecting your NF-kB negatively, you can affect it positively.

CAPEL'S HYPOTHESIS

Stress increases NF-kB-activity, but meditation and stress-reducing methods bring it back down to a healthy basic level. IL-6 production, for example—which depends on NF-kB—is substantially lower after a stress stimulus in people who meditate. Meditation is not a soft, esoteric activity, but it can penetrate deeply into the core of our cells and influence how our DNA functions.

One of the many examples of this is seen in the research into telomeres. This research was awarded the Nobel Prize for Medicine in 2009. Telomeres are the outer ends of the chromosomes. The telomeres become shorter each time the cell divides, and partly determine the lifespan of the cell. Because of stress, chromosomes shorten more quickly. The researchers turned the question around and explored whether telomeres lengthened again as a result of meditation—allowing a cell to live longer. They discovered that this is indeed the case.

Meditation can have a significant effect on important transcription factors, including NF-kB. It can also change the pH of the body. Wim Hof's concentrated breathing exercises can also be understood as a form of meditation, with the associated effects.

The combination of breathing, meditation and cold training changes the normal stress response to cold and to hypo- and hyperventilation. The normal stress response comprises the immediate release of adrenaline, followed by the production of stress hormones from the pituitary gland in the brain. These stress hormones trigger the production of cortisol by the adrenal glands. Cortisol has a strong impact on our bodies and also controls many functions, including the stimulation of NF-kB activity. However, Hof and his trained group clearly respond to stress differently. This different response is possibly due to the increased pH levels from the special breathing, and the resulting absence of pain and fear. The part of the brain normally stimulated by cold-induced pain is not activated. It does not send a signal—or perhaps it sends a different signal—to the pituitary gland, to change the stress response.

When Hof and his group started the special breathing exercises, a lot of adrenaline was released. Adrenaline is produced in response to hypo- or hyperventilation, and to cold. During the training, breathing and cold had become associated to each other. This association generated a conditioned response, as with nineteenth century Russian scientist Pavlov's dogs.

Pavlov noticed that the dogs would start salivating at the sight of food. He started ringing a bell when he gave the dogs food, so they would associate the sound of the bell with food. Soon, they started salivating when they heard the sound of the bell, even when there was no food. This process, known as conditioning, is very well known. It is very possible that Hof and his group produced extremely high levels of adrenaline as soon as they started their special breathing exercises—before they got into the ice bath—as a conditioned response.

The Wim Hof Method could be based on dissociating the sensations of pain and cold, changing the normal stress response. An altered stress response will directly impact the balance of transcription factors—and therefore hundreds of bodily functions. The high adrenaline production gives the advantages of acute stress, increasing our performance without the heightened NF-kB activity that normally accompanies it.

Given the relationship between high NF-kB activity and a large number of diseases, including the development of cancer, the WHM could have far-reaching consequences.

Scientists from various disciplines are working to unravel and understand Wim Hof's method. In January 2015, doctor and researcher Geert Buijze started a study known as the Cool Challenge. The results of the study will be interesting, as they could show the benefits from simply taking cold showers—instead of ice baths. Buijze started taking cold showers after going to Kilimanjaro with Hof. Ever since then, he has not been sensitive to the cold and hasn't been sick for a single day. As a scientist at the Academic Medical Centre in Amsterdam, Buijze knows that anecdotal evidence is not the same as hard facts. So, he decided to start the Cool Challenge with more than 3,000 volunteers. He divided the participants into four groups: the control group continued to take warm showers, another group took a cold shower for 30 seconds after showering normally, another group the same for 60 seconds, and the last for 90 seconds. They all answered the same questionnaire, which asked questions about the number of days they were ill. You can follow the results of current challenges on www.coolchallenge.nl.

People like Pickkers, Muskiet and Capel also continue to work on understanding the details of the WHM. In the coming years, much more will become clear and many new questions will arise. Every time we discover something about how our bodies work, new questions also emerge. The same will happen in the quest to fully understand the effects of cold exposure and breathing exercises. As we discover new knowledge, what we know now might be discarded in six month's time. In that sense, scientists are just like everyone else—they sometimes contradict themselves.

Bold claims—supported by scientific evidence—have been made. But, are they useful? Can we say that people with cancer can benefit from Wim Hof's method? No, we can't. Absolutely not. We just don't know exactly how cells, genes and transcription factors respond to the WHM. The material is too complex and our knowledge still insufficient. But we also can't say that people with cancer cannot benefit from these simple techniques.

The WHM is not dangerous—and imagine the possibility that it works. It is important to remember that the average person does not exist, and science only compares groups. Therefore, it does not prove how things will or will not work for a specific individual.

What can we say for certain about the impact of breathing exercises and cold on serious diseases? Saying nothing at all doesn't feel right. With this knowledge, we feel a sense of duty to share it widely. But being overly positive doesn't feel right, either. We don't want to give anyone false hope. On top of it all, we still don't know exactly how it works.

The following chapter will provide more background information on specific diseases, and will describe the WHM experiences of some who have suffered from those diseases. Again, we don't want to give people false hope, but these experiences might inspire you to see how the breathing exercises and cold might be able to help you—whether you are ill or in perfect health.

Who Can Benefit from the Wim Hof Method?

Now you know what the Wim Hof Method entails and what scientific studies have discovered about it. The next question is, who can benefit from it? We have already mentioned a number of diseases, such as rheumatism, obesity and Lyme disease. Trying the WHM with other diseases may also be worth it.

Before we describe a number of diseases and give examples of people who have started working with breathing exercises and cold training, we would first like to show how the WHM can help perfectly healthy people.

HEALTHY PEOPLE

No one in their right mind would take cold showers to stay healthy. If you are in perfect health, you're simply not concerned about being ill—or even the possibility that you might get ill.

But, there is still every reason for healthy people to take cold showers, or swim outside in cold water. It gives you the feeling that you are alive. Really alive. Especially if you have a job that requires sitting down most of the time. Even if the job is fine, you might not exactly spring out of bed every morning excited about getting to work. Taking a cold shower is a great start to the day. You will find yourself bursting with energy.

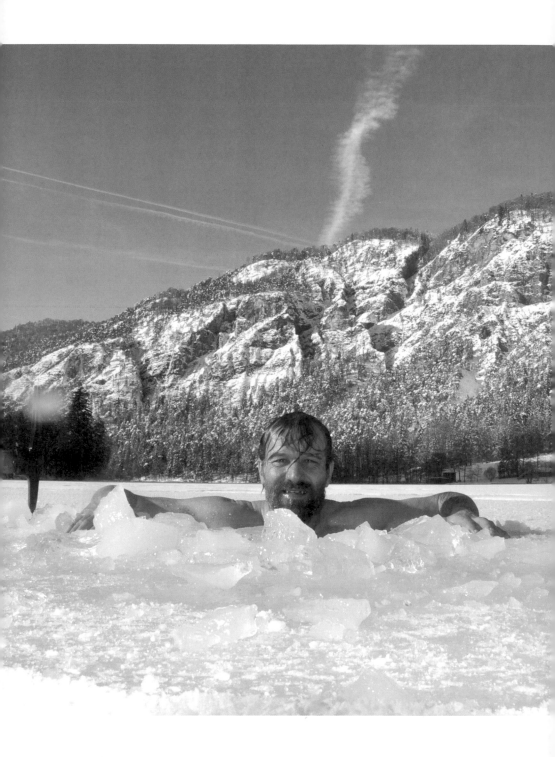

ATHLETES

Dutch champion skater Sven Kramer takes an ice bath after heavy training sessions to recover more quickly. After heavy training or a race, athletes' muscles produce substances like lactate that can stay in the body for a long time. Athletes want to get rid of surplus lactate as quickly as possible, so that they can start intensive training again without delay. Strenuous physical exercise also causes microscopic damage to the muscles. If you rest sufficiently, that damage is repaired and the body becomes stronger. This process is known as supercompensation. Hydrotherapy—sitting in an ice bath—speeds up the process of removing waste materials from the body. First, the blood vessels constrict, then when you get out of the ice bath, circulation resumes more actively. Research into the effect of a cold bath or alternate hot and cold baths shows that athletes' muscles are less stiff the following day.

Bleakly et al. conducted a large-scale literature study of the effects of cold-water baths on the body's ability to recover. Of the 58 studies they examined, they only found 17 good enough to explore in more detail. They compared cold baths with warm baths and passive recovery. One study compared cold baths and active recovery—running at an easy pace for 15 minutes. The results showed that 24 hours after the physical activity, athletes who took a cold bath experienced less muscle pain than those who had passively recovered.

After this brief look at healthy people and athletes, we will now describe the WHM in relation to a number of diseases and other health problems. Again, we would like to emphasize that this information is not intended to encourage you to stop regular treatments. It is also not intended to undermine or judge "conventional" medical treatment. But, we do want to encourage you to understand the link between the effect of breathing on the billions of cells in our bodies and possibly health problems or disorders.

Blood Pressure

The heart pumps the blood through the arteries, which generates pressure on the blood vessels. If this pressure rises too high, it increases the risks of cardiovascular disease. Doctors measure two values when testing the blood pressure: the higher (systolic) level and the lower (diastolic) level. Blood pressure is expressed in terms of these two levels; normal blood pressure is considered to be a systolic level of 120 mmHg (millimeters of mercury) and a diastolic level of 80 mm/Hg.

People with high blood pressure rarely notice any symptoms, but the continuous pressure on the blood vessels can cause damage to the organs and other structures including the heart muscles, arteries, eyes, kidneys, and brain.

The systolic level is the most variable and is particularly responsive to stress. But, the diastolic pressure is a good indication of cardiovascular disease risk. If the diastolic pressure is above 95 mmHg, doctors will prescribe a course of treatment. They will also advise the patient to give up smoking, eat a healthier diet, consume less salt, lose weight, get at least half an hour's physical activity a day, and learn how to manage stress. If all of those lifestyle changes do not help, the next step is to prescribe medication.

We feel it is a shame that doctors do not include exposure to cold in their advice. As seen in the chapter on cold training, you can train your blood vessels by exposing them to cold. Blood vessels contract in response to cold to secure the supply of blood to the vital organs. They open again when the body warms up. You can train them by closing them forcefully in response to cold and then opening them again by leaving the cold.

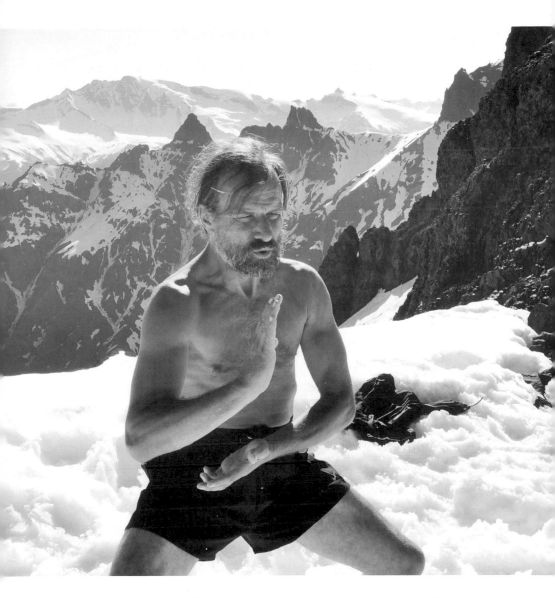

If you have high blood pressure, it seems to be something good to try. Of course, start by taking cold showers—do not jump straight in to an ice bath. It certainly helped Jack Egberts' mother (also described in the chapter on cold training). After taking cold showers for a month, and after consulting with her doctor, she was able to stop taking her medication.

CANCER

The reason we are discussing cancer in this book is because of Capel's ideas on NF-kB described in the previous chapter. To put it mildly, it is a little sensitive to talk about cancer in a book by Wim Hof on the importance of cold training and breathing exercises. As a friend of mine said very succinctly, "You're writing a book with Wim Hof? Isn't that the guy who says he can cure cancer just with breathing exercises and cold showers?"

Wim has never claimed he can cure cancer. He would never say that.

Yet my friend's hair stands on end when he hears the name Wim Hof. We hear reactions like this quite often—people who dismiss Wim as someone who gives people false hope.

Wim Hof says that he does not cure cancer. Yet astronaut and physicist Wubbo Ockels, who suffered from kidney cancer, started swimming in the cold water of the canals in Amsterdam after a week with Hof. And Dutch Philosopher Laureate René Gude (bone cancer) started doing Wim's breathing exercises. And journalist Mark Bos (prostate cancer) has a "cold seat" in his shed, a sort of wooden tub that you can sit in where the temperature is constantly 1°C (33.8°F).

Were these men desperately searching for a cure? On a leading Dutch current affairs television program, Ockels said that his American doctor had given him a year to live at maximum. But Ockels did not accept that. He said that he wanted to use the strength of his mind to make his body strong. He was looking for the primal human within himself, and said he was grateful to the cancer for giving him the opportunity to learn a lot more and meet so many new people. Ockels wanted to cure himself completely, but he died on May 18, 2014.

The evening before Ockels died, national newspaper reporter Arno Gelder visited him in the hospital. He wrote of the meeting: We shook each other's hands. He took off his oxygen mask. "Hello, Wubbo," I said. I was at a loss for words, but Ockels was alert and happy that I'd come to see him. "I've got a statement," he said. "For your readers. We have to work towards a new religion, a new energy. And it's called Humanity! It's all on the desktop of my computer. Martin will send it to you."

Gelder asked him whether he was afraid. "Of death? No, not at all. I've had a great life, a fantastic life. But it is terrible for Joos and the children. That is what troubles my soul the most..."

Ockels fought until the last moment. He couldn't beat his own disease, but he had the strength and energy to inspire others right up to the end.

Journalist and documentary maker Mark Bos is also fighting his illness. He described finding out about Wim Hof after he was diagnosed with cancer, and what he is doing with his knowledge of the WHM.

Bos learned he had prostate cancer in September, 2012. His prostate was seriously enlarged and the cancer had spread to his pubic bone. He was told that the cancer was inoperable. After this diagnosis, he underwent further tests at the Radboud University Medical Centre and received more bad news. The cancer had also spread to his liver, and was untreatable. Because of unpleasant side effects, Bos refused injections, but did take pills and set out on a quest. He started investigating his own disease, as though it were an interesting topic for a documentary.

He also started to do more physical activities and eat a healthier diet. He instinctively felt that it was a good time to do everything he considered healthy—but which he never had time for as a journalist. In any case, he wanted to do something.

By way of studying neuro-linguistic programming (NLP), he discovered the book *Quantum Healing* by Deepak Chopra. He also became acquainted with psychotherapy and Wim Hof. This was a logical consequence of his quest.

Bos tries to see his cancer as a companion—one that might always be with him. Yet, his ultimate wish is to be cured. Cold training and breathing exercises play an important role in his efforts to keep himself as physically fit and as positive as possible with healthy living. After the first training with Wim Hof, he was very enthusiastic about the effects. He had more energy and his mood was very positive for several days. So he decided to continue training with Wim Hof. He went to Poland for a week to do cold training in the mountains and did breathing exercises for more than an hour each day. The results were promising. After a scan in hospital, he heard good news. To the doctors' surprise, there was no sign of the cancer in his bones anymore.

Now that the cancer was no longer spreading, the doctors said that there was a small chance of curing it by removing the affected glands, followed by a seven-week course of radiation therapy. At first, Bos wasn't very enthusiastic, but he didn't want to put his fate in the hands of faith healers and die without having been treated. So he agreed to the operation.

It was not a success. The doctors removed 41 glands, 17 of which proved to be affected by cancer. But the tumor in his prostate proved too large. The radiation therapists cancelled the planned course of treatment (35 sessions in seven weeks) because they felt that it would not do any good. Bos was back at square one. He had undergone a serious operation for nothing. He was completely exhausted and disillusioned. He had to get his confidence in his recovery back—and that is what he did.

Just before his operation, Bos had decided to take part in the expedition to climb Kilimanjaro (see the chapter on commitment). His desire to get to the top was an enormous incentive to start working with the WHM again. He started training and improved his fitness. By December, 2013, he was able to run 19 kilometers again. But just as everything seemed to be going in the right direction again, Bos had to deal with yet another setback. His prostate-specific antigen (PSA), which had been 52 before the operation, had risen to 200 after the surgery and was now higher than 300. It was a disaster. Bos had to take it much easier with the training, and sustained an injury as well. But, he still went to Kilimanjaro. Through a combination of commitment and breathing exercises, he got to the top.

Bos has never believed that the WHM could cure him. But, he has noticed that it gives him extra energy every day so he can live his life more positively and more actively.

Considering the circumstances, he feels great. He runs, does breathing exercises, and cold training every day. Instead of lying in bed ill with prostate cancer, he lives his life to the fullest. He has a new girlfriend, and travels a lot. He has made a documentary about his illness, his quest and his experiences. It is called *Retour Hemel, A Return Ticket to Heaven*.

Does he have advice for people with cancer?

"No," Bos says, "Not for fellow cancer patients. My story is an example of how you can improve your life circumstances yourself. But I do have some advice for the doctors who treat us: they should come out of their straitjackets of guidelines and protocols and show a little more interest in how people who do it their own way achieve real progress."

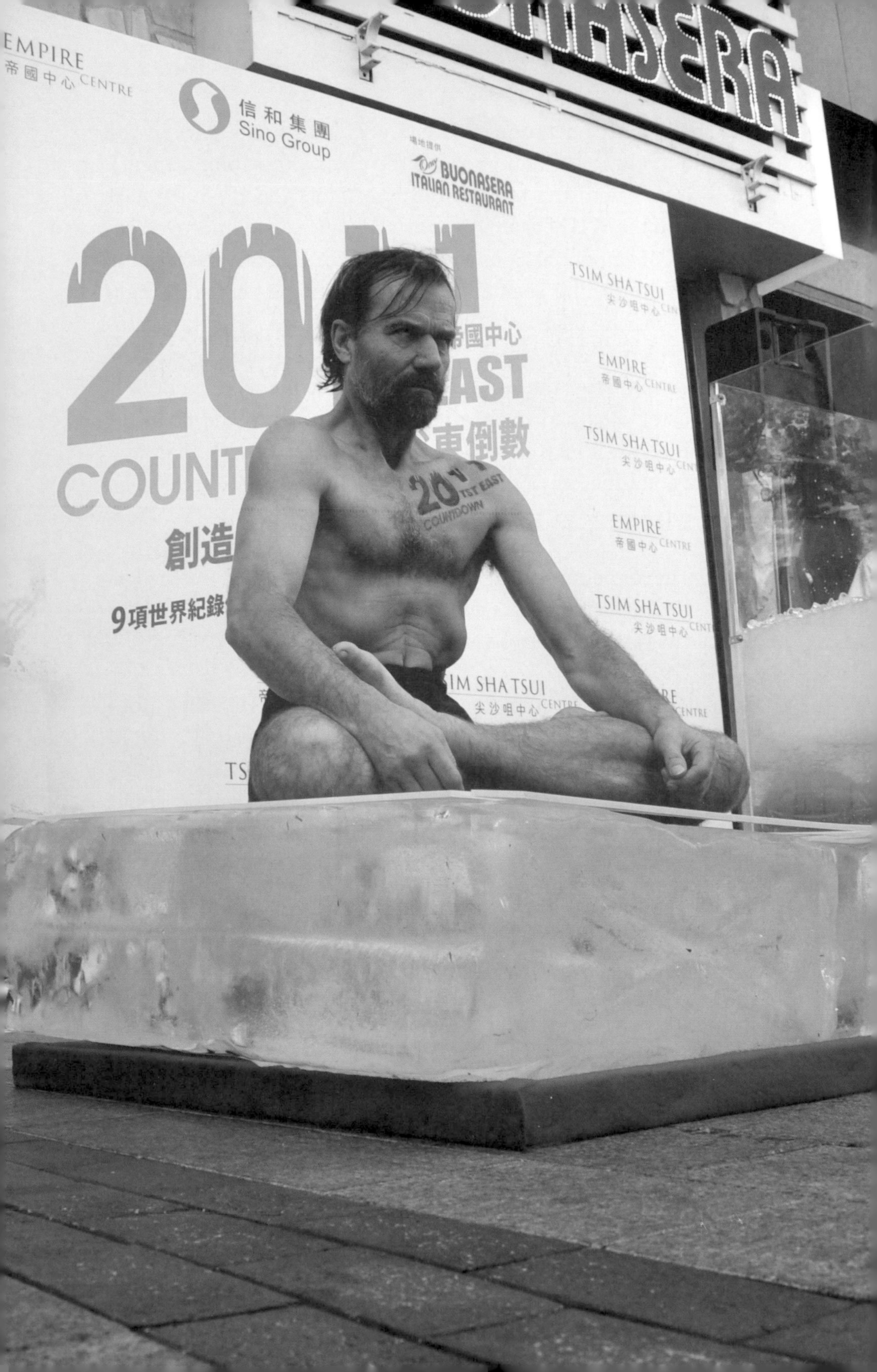
EMPIRE
帝國中心 CENTRE
信和集團
Sino Group
BUONASERA
ITALIAN RESTAURANT
TSIM SHA TSUI
EMPIRE
帝國中心 CENTRE
TSIM SHA TSUI
EMPIRE
帝國中心 CENTRE
TSIM SHA TSUI
9項世界紀錄

INFLAMMATION

As described earlier in the chapter on science, it is interesting to observe what happens with diseases where inflammation plays an important role. Pickkers discovered that Wim Hof is capable of controlling his inflammatory proteins. Could this be meaningful for people who take anti-inflammatory medications? As we said before, the people tested in Hof's group were healthy. So, we do not have any tested information about the WHM and its effects on people who are sick. We don't know whether people who take anti-inflammatory medication could benefit from it. But, it is a proven fact that people can control their own inflammatory proteins. So the same may be true for those who take drugs to control inflammation. These medications are not always successful and can have serious side effects.

The four main types of anti-inflammatory drugs:

- Corticosteroids are adrenal gland cortex hormones that stimulate the production of anti-inflammatory proteins. The most widely known corticosteroid is prednisone.

- Antibodies act on a specific protein and inhibit the inflammation that is linked to that protein. An example of an antibody is anti-TNF-α.

- Non-steroidal anti-inflammatory drugs (NSAIDs) relieve inflammation. Examples are aspirin and ibuprofen.

- Disease-modifying anti-rheumatic drugs (DMARDs) reduce tissue damage through reducing inflammation. An example of a DMARD is methotrexate.

The list of diseases and health problems linked to inflammation is growing rapidly as we gain new insights. The diseases include rheumatism, Crohn's disease, high blood pressure, obesity, insomnia, type II diabetes, Alzheimer's, depression, some forms of cancer, and fatigue.

We will look at a number of these diagnoses and—especially—see what patients have experienced.

RHEUMATISM

Rheumatism is a collective name for more than one hundred diseases. The most well known are rheumatoid arthritis, osteoarthritis, fibromyalgia, gout and Bechterew's disease. When doctors talk about rheumatism, they usually mean rheumatoid arthritis. Rheumatoid arthritis is an inflammation of the joints—the cause of this disease is unknown.

The American Rheumatism Association uses the following criteria for rheumatoid arthritis (five of the following must be present for at least six weeks):

- Morning stiffness
- Pain when moving at least one joint
- Swelling due to soft tissue thickening in at least one joint
- Swelling in soft tissue of at least one other joint
- Characteristic changes in synovial membrane
- Characteristic nodules on muscle or tendon

If rheumatism is diagnosed, it is usually treated with medication. Breathing exercises or exposure to cold are rarely applied—which is a shame, cold training can be an effective supplement to regular treatment.

Marianne Peper is an excellent example.

MARIANNE PEPER

I interviewed Marianne Peper at her house in Deurne. Before we started the interview, she wanted to show me something. She opened a plastic bag and tipped out eleven small boxes onto the table. The boxes contained these medicines:

- Omeprazole 40mg
- Prednisolone 20mg
- Levocetirizine 5mg
- Naproxen 250mg
- Plaquenil 200mg
- Clonidine 0,025mg
- Meloxicam
- Diclofenac
- Ventolin
- Paracetamol
- Seretide

Marianne used to take all of them. Additionally, she had a prednisone injection every three weeks. On October, 17, 2013, she decided to stop taking her medications. It was a strange thing to do, as Marianne has rheumatoid arthritis, fibromyalgia, several allergies and pain all over her body. She was in so much pain that she could not even dress herself.

And yet, she decided to stop her medication. Why?

She told me that her father died from taking prednisone. As a child, she used to go to see local football team FC Twente and they would sing the club song "One Day We'll be Champions" together. By the time FC Twente won the league in 2010, her father had already died. His early death still upsets Marianne. She didn't associate her medications with getting better, but with the death of her father. The medications only reduced the symptoms. That is why she decided to stop taking the medications in 2013. After she stopped taking them, she went through hell for a month and a half. She did take sleeping tablets, otherwise she wouldn't have been able to stick it out.

Pain, pain, and more pain.

It was also a difficult time for her husband. He took care of her, helped her dress, took over a lot of the housework and stood by his wife. His humor helped to lighten the load during this period, but it was still tough. If he even touched Marianne it hurt, so they were unable to make love.

Then she saw Wim Hof on television. Intuitively she thought that Wim could help her. Hof said that we are capable of much more than we think. Marianne wanted to know more, so Wim came to their house to explain the breathing exercises.

Marianne started doing the exercises and felt a lot better after the first week. She went to Poland for a week. Along with the breathing exercises, she also trained with exposure to extreme cold. She stepped into an ice-cold stream (just above freezing point) and walked to the top of a mountain in the snow in short trousers. By the end of the week, she felt reborn. At home, she made a special bath in the garden to continue training in the cold.

It all sounds too good to be true, but Marianne emphasizes that it takes a lot of hard work. She does breathing exercises every day and takes an ice bath at least twice a week. If she doesn't do it, the pain comes back immediately. Yet, she is delighted.

Her rheumatologist had advised her to get an infrared lamp and take medication. But Wim Hof taught her about the benefits of cold, and now she no longer needs medication. She now refuses to call herself a patient. Her husband agrees, with a contented wink.

CROHN'S DISEASE

We also have an exceptional story to tell about Crohn's disease. Crohn's disease is a chronic disease of the stomach and the intestines that affects about 20,000 people in the Netherlands. Mostly, it affects the large or small intestines. The inflammation reduces the absorption of some nutrients in the small intestine, leading to loss of weight and nutrient deficiencies. This also causes fatigue and a wide variety of non-specific health problems. The inflammation can also cause permanent damage to the wall of the intestines, resulting in blood loss.

The problems are not restricted to the intestines. People with Crohn's disease often also have pain in their joints and skin diseases. Sometimes, sections of the intestine have to be removed to keep the disease under control.

However, there is evidence that the Wim Hof Method can keep the disease at bay.

MATHIJS STORM

In 2008, Mathijs Storm was diagnosed with Crohn's disease. He was relieved to finally have a diagnosis. He had been suffering from fatigue for many years. After work, he would just collapse in exhaustion on the couch. He could never really indulge his love of martial arts because his system was too weak. But, after a visit to the doctor and a referral to the hospital he knew why— he had Crohn's disease.

Storm has a humorous way of describing his disease. "I have an extreme right-wing intestinal wall," he says. "It attacks everything that is foreign, and that leads to inflammation."

He was prescribed drugs to inhibit the inflammation. Most of them had no effect. Only a few heavy-duty medicines from the TNF-α group—biological agents—seemed to bring some relief. Storm learned to live with the disease. He identified with it since it explained his fatigue and limitations.

But after two years, something started to gnaw at him. Was he self-imposing more restrictions than necessary? Of course Crohn's disease is Crohn's disease, but there are many ways to generate more energy—even with chronic intestinal inflammation. He started reading books about breathing, fitness, and nutrition. He also started meditating. In his quest for more knowledge and information, he found Wim Hof's website and watched a few video clips.

He was immediately enthusiastic about the benefits of the breathing techniques, but didn't think Hof's cold training was appropriate for him. Then, more than a year later, his brother-in-law told him that Wim only eats once a day. This encouraged him to take another look at Wim's website. Maybe chronic inflammation of the intestines could be relieved by eating less.

On the website, Storm read that the results of medical research cautiously suggested that Wim could use his method to influence his immune system. Storm was fascinated.

He decided to attend one of Wim's workshops to see whether the WHM could help him. Storm accidentally registered for an instructor's weekend, rather than a regular workshop. But, he still took part in everything—the breathing exercises and sitting in an ice bath. After the weekend, he was delighted and bursting with energy.

Storm regained control over his body. For the whole weekend, he had not felt like a patient. Back home, he started doing the exercises and his mood improved. In the evenings after work, he had the time and energy to do odd jobs around the house. His energy levels continued to rise sharply, and he even started cycling back and forth to work, which he had not been able to do before.

These experiences inspired him to do more. Storm continued with the instructor's course and gained more and more control over his body. Then, out of the blue, Wim Hof asked him if he wanted to climb Kilimanjaro. "What?" Storm thought, "Isn't that a 6,000-meter (3.7 mile) high mountain in Tanzania?" For a long time, Storm doubted that the trip was a good idea before he decided to go. During the training, his confidence in his abilities grew even more. He cycled to work in the mornings bare-chested—even in temperatures only a few degrees above freezing. One morning, the police pulled him over and asked if he was feeling ok. When he explained that he was going to climb Kilimanjaro with Wim Hof and was doing cold training, the officers laughed and wished him good luck. They had already heard about Wim through local hero Henk van den Bergh, who also worked with the WHM and barely had any more problems with his rheumatism.

The expedition to Kilimanjaro was tough, but Storm made it to the top and was delighted. A month later, he had surprising news from the hospital—they hadn't found any more indications of inflammation in his stools. Storm was convinced this was because of the breathing exercises and the cold training.

Later, Storm learned that he had to keep doing the exercises. In his enthusiasm about having so much more energy, he started doing too much. He started working harder and renovating his house. He also devoted a lot of attention to his wife, who was heavily pregnant. All of this left him too little time to do the exercises and his inflammation levels increased again. The Crohn's disease came back. When it was first discovered in 2008, Storm was happy to find an explanation for his problems when he was officially diagnosed as a Crohn's patient. Now, he was happy because he knew what he had to do. Now, he knew how to combat the inflammation: he needed to get back to "Hoffing".

In the period that followed, he once again felt he had control over his body—he was not dependent only on doctors and drugs. His doctor responded positively to this development and emphasized the importance of balance in our lives. The Wim Hof Method helps Storm maintain that balance and gives him the strength to stay in control of his life.

He might have Crohn's disease, but Storm is no longer a patient.

DEPRESSION

It is well known that people with autoimmune diseases suffer from persistent inflammatory reactions, when the immune system attacks a body's own tissue. In the 1980s, immunologist Hemmo Drexhage noticed something remarkable. Behavioral disorders like autism and schizophrenia proved to be surprisingly common among people with autoimmune diseases.

It occurred to Drexhage that persistent inflammatory responses could also affect the brain. Initially, his ideas did not receive much support from psychiatrists, but nowadays they are increasingly taking his theory seriously.

In an interesting article in *NWT Magazine,* journalist Jop de Vrieze wrote that in recent years, psychiatric disorders—especially depression, autism and schizophrenia—have been increasingly linked to the immune system. It is claimed that they are caused by dormant inflammations disrupting the normal functioning of the brain. One indication is that psychiatric patients have higher concentrations of cytokines—signaling molecules for the immune system—in their blood and brains.

The immune system works differently in the brain than in the rest of the body. The brain has its own immune cells, known as microglia. They are activated when the brain is under a threat. At least, that is how they are supposed to work. Someone suffering from psychiatric disorders like depression, may have microglia in a permanent state of readiness. That is a disastrous situation. Microglia are responsible for the brain's resistance to threats, and they also maintain links between neurons. They break these links or create new ones as necessary, but they cannot do everything at the same time. So if they are activated to respond to a threat, they cannot also maintain the links between neurons. As a result of long term permanent readiness, the links within the brain can function less efficiently. You can compare microglia to traffic controllers who make sure the traffic runs smoothly. If a traffic controller is attacked by a wasp and he tries to chase it away, he can no longer regulate the traffic, which will become chaotic. It is therefore important for your brain that the microglia are not continually occupied trying to combat real or imaginary threats.

The Netherlands is officially one of the happiest countries in the world. Yet nearly a million people in the Netherlands take anti-depressants. While anti-depressants combat depression, they are also prescribed to treat anxiety or compulsive disorders. This paradox inspired Trudy Dehue to write a book, *De Depressie-epidemie* (The Depression Epidemic).

In her book, Dehue expresses reservations about the effectiveness of pills and is critical of the triumphant mood of the 1980s when Prozac was heralded as the pharmaceutical answer to depression. After all, what do we know about depression? Is it caused by personal experiences that result in despondency and apathy? Or is it a stand-alone disorder caused by disruptions in our hormones or neurotransmitters? It may be triggered by unpleasant experiences, but not necessarily in every case.

The extent to which breathing exercises and cold training can help alleviate depression or help people to recover from it will need to be researched more closely in the coming years. Wim Hof is currently working with a large number of psychiatrists to investigate what approach works, possibly in combination with medication.

ASTHMA

Just as high levels of inflammation play an important role in rheumatism, Crohn's disease, and perhaps in depression, an inflamed epithelium—the layer of cells that line the airways—is also important in relation to asthma.

Konstantin Buteyko, the Ukrainian doctor and scientist already mentioned in the chapter on breathing, said, "No deep breathing, no asthma". We understand what happens in the body during an asthma attack, but doctors are still in the dark about why people get asthma in the first place. According to the World Health Organization, there are between 100 and 150 million asthma patients in the world. In the Netherlands, some 430,000 people have been officially diagnosed by their doctors as suffering from asthma. Currently, asthma is mainly tackled by treating the symptoms. Drugs like Ventolin ensure that the patient gets air quickly, but these drugs do not cure the problem.

Buteyko claimed to have discovered the real cause of asthma: a response to chronic—often unconscious—hyperventilation. If you suffer from chronic hyperventilation, the body loses too much carbon dioxide (see the chapter on breathing). Carbon dioxide plays an important role in a wide variety of processes in the body, including the absorption of oxygen by muscles and organs.

When someone breathes too much for an extended period, the body protests and tries to prevent further loss of carbon dioxide by making it more difficult to exhale. One way the body can do this is to tense up the muscles around the airways. This is what happens during an asthma attack. Buteyko sees asthma as one of the body's defense mechanisms, an attempt to prevent further loss of carbon dioxide.

Dick Kuiper, founder of the Dutch Buteyko Institute, wrote a book about this titled *Leven onder astma* (Living with Asthma). Breathing expert Stans van der Poel also agrees on the importance of sufficient carbon dioxide.

What happens in the lungs during an asthma attack?

In his book, Kuiper explains that three changes occur:

1. The airways—the supply and waste-removal pipes of our breathing system—cramp. The airways are surrounded by smooth muscle tissue and run deep into the lungs, continually supplying the alveoli with fresh air. During an asthma attack, this smooth muscle tissue can cramp up. This can happen in the upper part of the lungs, but may also occur much deeper. For example, the cramping can also happen close to the alveoli. The airways then become constricted, making breathing more difficult.

2. Inflamed epithelium. The airways are covered with a thin layer of cells called the epithelium. The epithelium can become inflamed in response to chemicals that we breathe in for example. The epithelium swells up which makes breathing more difficult.

3. Increased mucus production. The epithelium comprises cells that produce mucous and cilia cells, which together ensure that the lungs remain clean and sterile. The mucous captures dust and bacilli that cover the inside wall of the airways, while the cilia transport the mucous away towards the throat. During an asthma attack, the epithelium can produce so much extra mucous that the cilia have difficulty removing it. Again, this makes breathing more difficult.

With asthma, the main focus is on inflammation of the airways. With this in mind, professor of clinical chemistry, Frits Muskiet's response to the tests at the Radboud UMC is especially interesting: "Because of our current lifestyles, we live with a permanent low level of infection. You could say that we are chronically infected, but because it is so low, we don't feel it at all. We don't notice it, but is the breeding ground of many diseases. Wim Hof's group has shown us that it is possible to repress that inflammatory response."

If one of the main physical changes during an asthma attack is inflammation of the airways, and we know that asthma sufferers (people who use a short-acting β2-adrenergic agonist to dilate the airways more than three times a week) are advised to take anti-inflammatory drugs, then the Wim Hof Method could achieve the same result with fewer side effects. Konstantin Buteyko emphasizes the importance of more shallow breathing and says that breathing in through the nose is sufficient to ensure that you do not breathe too deeply.

Wim Hof's breathing techniques, which involve breathing in deeply and then exhaling slowly, seem to be completely at odds with this. Yet, after doing these exercises, most people start to breathe more calmly, and their carbon dioxide levels return to normal. The big difference is that during the exercises, your breathing is controlled. People with asthma breathe too deeply and cannot control it.

ARTHRITIS

Since 2013, arthritis has been associated with inflammation. Arthritis is a progressive disease in which the cartilage between the joints steadily erodes causing pain and stiffness. Some 1.2 million people in the Netherlands suffer from some form of arthritis. Current treatment involves taking painkillers. If the case is very serious, patients may be surgically fitted with a new joint. For a long time, arthritis was believed to be a disease of the cartilage itself, caused by wear and tear on the joints. That observation is consistent with the fact that arthritis often occurs in older people, and obese people whose knee joints wear more quickly because of the extra weight. This sounds plausible except that obese people often have arthritis in their hands, which cannot be explained by an excessive mechanical burden.

On June 18, 2013, Lobke Gierman (1983) was awarded a PhD for his dissertation, *Inflammation: a link between metabolic syndrome and osteoarthritis?* After the research, Gierman said, "We now have a completely different view of arthritis. A mild inflammatory response, caused by being overweight, is probably significant, especially in the early stages of the disease."

TYPE-II DIABETES

There are two types of diabetes.

Characteristics of type 1 diabetes:

- The body hardly produces any insulin
- The body's immune system accidentally destroys the cells that produce insulin
- Patients have to inject themselves with insulin a few times a day, or use an insulin pump
- Type 1 diabetes used to be called "juvenile diabetes"
- 1 in 10 people with diabetes have type 1

Characteristics of type 2 diabetes:

- The body is resistant to insulin
- The body no longer responds to insulin properly (insulin insensitivity)
- Excess weight, lack of physical activity, age, and a history of the disease in the family can increase the risk of contracting type 2 diabetes
- Patients are usually treated with drugs, advised on a healthy diet and the importance of physical activity. Sometimes they also have to inject insulin
- Formerly called "adult-onset diabetes", but now it is quite common among younger people
- 9 out of 10 people with diabetes have type 2

Recently, there has been greater attention to the link between obesity and type 2 diabetes, and between these two factors and inflammation.

The Dutch Diabetes Fund website has the following message:

Obesity plays an important role in the development of type 2 diabetes, because the body responds less well to insulin in people who are overweight. There are strong indications that inflammation of fat tissue also plays a role, and research has been conducted to study this link further.

The research showed that the protein cytokine IL-1 plays an important role in the inflammation of fat tissue. This was studied in the cells of test animals and humans. The protein is more active in the case of obesity, especially in fat around the waist. With mice, the body responded better to insulin when the protein was inhibited.

The researchers also discovered a sister protein to IL-1, IL-37, which has the opposite effect. In test animals, IL-37 provided protection against both inflammation and insulin insensitivity in the case of obesity. This may offer a new way to tackle type 2 diabetes.

These results make it possible, in the future, to explore whether the inflammation can be inhibited with drugs, with the ultimate aim of improving insulin insensitivity.

The above statement is yet another an indirect link between inflammation and a disease of prosperity. More research is sure to follow. There is good reason to give cold training and breathing exercises a fair chance in this research. Although we do not yet know what comes first—the inflammation, the obesity or diabetes—it is certainly worth investigating.

How are inflammation and obesity related?

OBESITY

There is increasing evidence that obesity and inflammation are related. In 2013, research in Brisbane, Australia, showed that obese people have abnormal levels of the inflammatory protein PAR2 in their abdominal fat tissue. The research—published in *The FASEB Journal*—was conducted by David P. Fairlie, PhD. Fairlie conducted tests on obese rats and humans. The results offer new insights into the link between inflammation and obesity. The level of protein PAR2 even increased on the surfaces of human immune cells from exposure to normal fatty acids in the diet. Obese rats that were fed a lot of sugar and fat had high levels of PAR2. But if they were given an oral drug that binds to PAR2, the inflammation caused by the protein was blocked. The same applied to the other negative effects from a high-fat and high-sugar diet.

> *"This important new finding links obesity and high fat, high sugar diets with changes in immune cells and inflammatory status, highlighting an emerging realization that obesity is an inflammatory disease," said Fairlie, who is based at the Institute for Molecular Bioscience at the University of Queensland. "Drugs designed to block certain inflammatory proteins, as in this report, may be able to prevent and treat obesity, which in turn is a major risk factor for type 2 diabetes, heart disease, stroke, kidney failure, limb amputation, and cancers."*

Gerald Weissmann, M.D., Editor-in-Chief of *The FASEB Journal*, added, "We know that eating too much and not exercising enough makes you overweight, and then obese, but why? The bottom line of this report is that obesity is an inflammatory disease, and inflammation plays a greater role in the downward spiral to obesity than most people realize. It appears that once we can control the inflammation, we can begin to get everything else in line. Fortunately, these scientists have already identified one promising compound that seems to work."

The Australian research is interesting. But, the researchers' conclusion that drugs be used to control inflammatory proteins needs to be considered against the documented benefits of breathing exercises and cold training. Instead, why not try changing the diet, adding more physical activity, breathing exercises and cold training? That can also possibly control inflammatory proteins.

Annemarie Heuvel discovered that result herself. Heuvel, a former top water polo player, now owns a company called TopsportConnect. After she gave up top-level sports, she devoted all her energy to her new enterprise. That meant a lot of meetings, traveling, and a lot of eating. As a result, she put on a lot of weight. For many years she tried a succession of diets, but never with the desired results—until former teammate Marianne Peper got her interested in the Wim Hof Method. She completely changed her lifestyle and by combining a healthy low-salt diet, drinking a lot of water, and the WHM, she has now lost 14 kilograms (31 pounds) and feels physically and mentally fit again.

Besides inflammation, brown fat is also an important factor. Brown fat tissue is mainly produced when two proteins (PRDM16 and BPM7) are activated in response to cold.

As we explained earlier, the body has two kinds of fat tissue: white and brown. White fat tissue is used to store energy, while babies and other mammals in particular use brown fat to maintain the right body temperature. It is actually strange that adult humans hardly have any more brown fat, since it is such a valuable source of fuel. In cold areas, people who still work outside a lot still have high levels of brown fat, as does Wim Hof.

Brown fat tissue is produced when your body is cold. It also ensures that your body maintains a good balance between stored fat and fat used as fuel. Unlike white fat tissue, brown fat tissue contains a lot of mitochondria. Mitochondria are the power plants of our bodies. They enable brown fat tissue to burn more fat than white fat tissue, which contains hardly any mitochondria.

In short, a cold body produces more brown fat tissue, which allows more fat to be burned in the cells. The more brown fat you have, the more fat you can burn—and the more weight you can lose.

In the context of energy and fat burning, it is also interesting to consider what may happen in the case of people who suffer from chronic fatigue.

FATIGUE

Former pulmonary function laboratory assistant Stans van der Poel's theory is also interesting in relation to our examination of the body's energy systems. In her book *Chronische vermoeidheid nooit meer* (No more chronic fatigue), she wrote that nutrients like fats, proteins and carbohydrates are burned at the cellular level. That energy is required by all the muscles and organs, when in use and at rest.

Like a normal fire, the burning process requires fuel and oxygen. Oxygen is inhaled with the air and absorbed by the lungs. It is then carried by the blood to every cell in the muscles and organs.

Adenosine triphosphate (ATP) is the body's primary energy source. When ATP is broken down, energy is released. ATP is a relatively large, heavy molecule, so it is impossible to store the body's entire energy requirement as ATP. The body has an efficient solution to this problem in the form of different energy systems, all of which supply energy in the form of ATP in a different way. Consequently, when we need energy, we can tap into five "storage pots", which all provide ATP in their own way:

- Fat
- Glucose (aerobic)
- Glycolysis (anaerobic)
- Creatine phosphate (CP)
- Free ATP

The body's energy requirement depends on the intensity of the activity. Each storage pot has a different capacity and availability. It is important to know that the different energy systems always work together, but that the relative contribution of each one varies, depending on the duration and intensity of the activity.

The less intense the activity, the more low-energy fats are used as fuel. More intense efforts make use of more free ATP. The energy generated is released by the breakdown of organic compounds. This process can take place with oxygen (aerobic) or without it (anaerobic).

The store of fat is—by far—the largest source of energy, even if you are not at all overweight. The body's fat reserves are designed for light, long-lasting activity, as the energy is released slowly. But when the body requires energy quickly (ATP), the aerobic processes are too slow and glucose will be broken down without oxygen. This chemical process, glycolysis, releases energy in a different way and is anaerobic.

In the case of extremely intense activity, your body makes use of the small quantities of free ATP and creatine phosphate (CP) stored in the muscles. They contain enough stored CP to supply sufficient energy for 10 to 30 seconds, and sufficient ATP for only a two to four second short burst of power.

Let's go back to fatigue.

Your body is using energy all day—even when at rest or engaged in little activity. Free ATP and CP are of little use for a whole day's work or for physical labor. Glucose and glycogen will keep you going for an hour, two at the most if you are a top-level athlete. As we have seen with people on hunger strikes, our bodies have enough fat to keep us alive for several days. A healthy body first burns the fat stored in the muscles and later taps into the subcutaneous fat reserves. When an intense activity stops, the fat in the muscles is replenished from fat tissue. The greater the effort, the more the body calls on its glucose reserves.

However, test results show that people suffering from chronic fatigue also tap into their sugar reserves, rather than their fat, while at rest. People who suffer from burn-out, chronic fatigue syndrome (CFS), Pfeiffer's disease, and fibromyalgia use energy as if they were constantly engaged in strenuous physical activity. So, while people suffering from fatigue feel that they are resting, their bodies are still hard at work. Their reserves are not being replenished and the body becomes exhausted. The body has become a sugar-burning machine. Although many CFS patients are not overweight, their body fat percentage is relatively high because their fat reserves are not being used. They even use their sugar reserves at night, which explains why they even feel exhausted in the morning.

Breathing is an important factor for the body being "on"—active rather than at rest. Van der Poel links this to a disrupted balance between oxygen and carbon dioxide in the blood. According to her research, a shortage of carbon dioxide in the blood raises the pH value. The carbon dioxide shortage is caused by breathing too rapidly or too deeply, which brings us back to Konstantin Buteyko and his ideas about asthma.

The breathing exercises and the possibility of mobilizing brown fat as a fuel can also have beneficial effects for people suffering from fatigue.

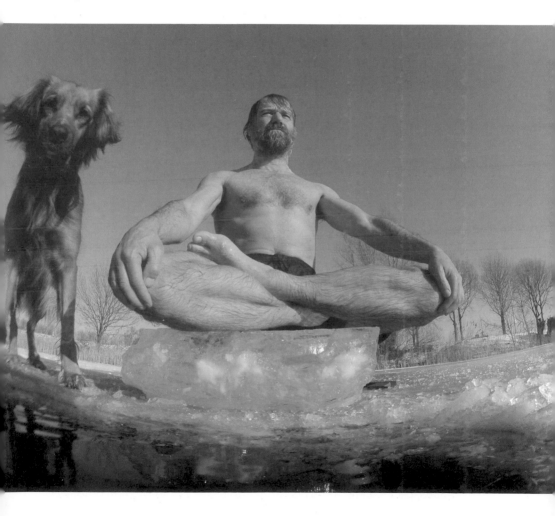

"TWITTER PROBLEMS"

When I was finishing this book, I posted a message on Twitter: "Finishing a book with @Iceman_Hof. Has anyone cured their health problems with the WHM and think it should be included in the book?"

Twitter is not my favorite medium, but I was interested to get any reactions about complaints or disorders that didn't emerge during the interviews and research I conducted for this book.

And, indeed, I did receive some reactions that I would like to share with you. They are not about serious diseases and I haven't checked on any of them with doctors, but they do come from enthusiastic users of the WHM. Since breathing exercises and cold training are not expensive drugs and have no severe side effects, you can easily try them out for yourself.

VARICOSE VEINS

Blue-purple blood vessels that show up through your skin are known as varicose veins. They can be small capillaries or large swollen veins visible as lumps. It is not completely clear why varicose veins develop, and it may be linked to a variety of factors.

The heart pumps blood through the arteries to all parts of the body and it returns to the heart through the veins. If you tense up your calf muscles, the blood vessels in your calf are pressed together. Because there are valves in the veins in your legs, the blood cannot flow downwards. Instead, it is pressed upwards towards your heart. When the blood from your legs does not flow back to your heart properly, it collects in your veins. The pressure in the veins increases, they dilate, and the valves no longer close properly. Badly functioning valves stop the blood from flowing upwards, so more blood accumulates in the veins and the veins dilate even further. Piles (hemorrhoids) are also varicose veins, but in and around the anus.

After my message on Twitter, I received a number of responses from people who were cured—completely unexpectedly—of their piles after practicing cold training.

COLD HANDS AND FEET

If you take cold showers, you will have fewer problems with cold hands and feet. It sounds a little contradictory, but it is actually very logical. After being exposed to extreme cold, your body will start to generate heat, just like switching on a thermostat. When the exposure to the cold stops—for example because you turned off the shower—your body continues to generate heat.

Besides cold training, breathing exercises also help you get rid of cold hands and feet. One cause of cold hands and feet can be irregular, rapid breathing. It sounds strange, but it really is true. If you breathe quickly, you will exhale too much carbon dioxide. The ratio of oxygen to carbon dioxide in your blood should be around 3:2; but if you breathe too fast, you disrupt this balance. With too little carbon dioxide in your body, your blood vessels contract, and your circulation is less efficient, which you will immediately notice in your extremities—your hands and feet.

THE SECRET TO A LONG LIFE

After my message on Twitter, someone sent me an article from the Dutch national newspaper *Algemeen Dagblad*, describing a study of the effects of ibuprofen. The headline said:

IBUPROFEN COULD BE THE SECRET OF A LONG LIFE

The researchers had tested ibuprofen—usually used to alleviate pain, fight fever, and reduce inflammation—on yeast, fungi and worms. Not exactly a study to get my heart beating faster, but the link—yet again—to an anti-inflammatory drug was interesting.

The drug seemed to significantly inhibit aging. Researchers at Texas A&M University and elsewhere gave yeast, worms and fungi a daily dose of ibuprofen for three years, comparable to a dose taken by humans. The life of yeast proved to be extended by 17%, or 12 years in human terms. The worms and flies also lived substantially longer, around 10%. They seemed to live their extra years in good health, too.

Ellen Nollen, professor of cell biology at the University Medical Centre in Groningen, called the results "promising". In an earlier study, ibuprofen was linked to reducing the risks of contracting aging diseases like Alzheimer's. "It clearly contains something that intervenes in the cell in a different way to other methods of prolonging life," Nollen said, adding "This is very much worth investigating further." Scientists say that a lot, but in this case, it seems like a valid suggestion.

COMBATING STRESS IN THE HERE AND NOW

"Exposure to the cold always brings me completely and intensely back to the here and now," wrote Léon Dantuma. "When I'm under stress or have a lot on my mind, I often take a cold shower. And I do the same when I'm tired to give me an energy shot." I saw a lot of responses with a similar message. More contact with your body, more relaxation, and less stress. It sounds logical, no matter how woolly it might seem. And it is an encouragement for healthy people to also give it a try.

Good health, shelter, food and drink. You might say that's all a person needs to be happy. Yet, there are thousands of people with a house, enough to eat and drink, and who are in good health, who spend the whole day agitated and flustered, their heads filled with everything they have to do. That is a great shame. Freshen yourself up, take a cold shower and see what it does for you.

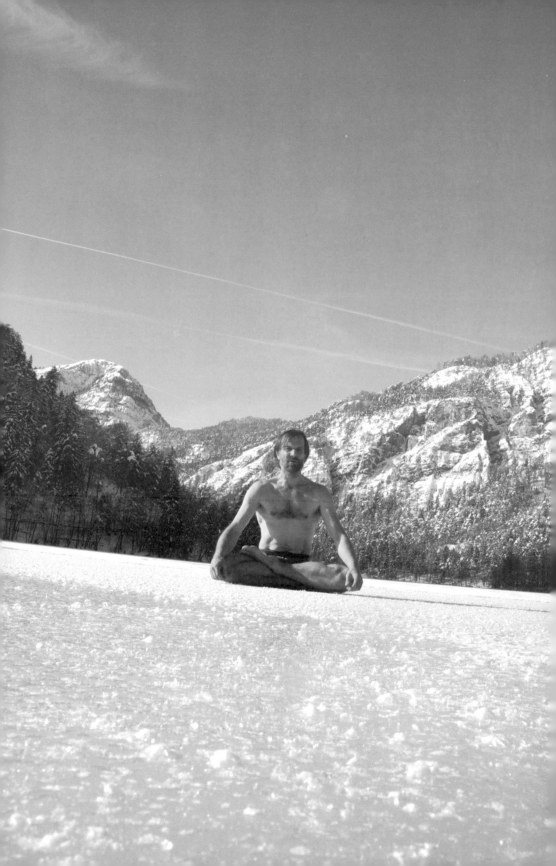

Do It Yourself in 30 Days—Getting Real and Taking Action

Reading a book is all well and good. But, it would be a shame if this knowledge were to remain at an intellectual level and you didn't take action.

We want to encourage you to really start working with the breathing exercises and cold training for 30 days.

Do this breathing exercise every day:

— **Breathe in deeply, and then exhale**
— **Breathe at the pace and rhythm that feel most comfortable**
— **Repeat 30 times**

On the last repetition, breathe out completely, then inhale again very deeply, exhale again slowly, and then hold the breath.

You want to breathe in deeply and out again slowly and without exerting pressure. By not fully exhaling, a small amount of air remains behind in the lungs. After breathing in and out 30 times, hold your breath after the last exhale, and wait until you feel the need to breathe in again. Practice this exercise until you feel tingling, light in the head, or sluggish.

You can check whether your body changes during the breathing exercises by measuring how long you can hold your breath. Time how long you can hold your breath before doing the exercises, and again afterwards. If you can hold your breath longer and longer, that is a good sign.

COLD SHOWERS

Take a warm shower, as you always do. Then, while the water is still warm, start doing breathing exercises. Breathe in and breathe out slowly. Do this a few times and then turn the shower to cold. Try to keep breathing calmly. Stay under the cold shower for a minute. In the second week, stay under the cold shower once for two minutes. In the third week, do the same once for three minutes. And in the fourth week, stay under the cold shower once for five minutes, without taking a warm shower first.

It is also good to give your hands and feet an ice bath once a week. Fill a bowl with cold water and add lumps of ice or ice cubes. If you don't have an ice-maker, you can buy ice cubes at the supermarket. Put your hands in the ice water for two minutes and then do the same with your feet.

Would you prefer to sit in an ice bath or swim outdoors in the winter? We certainly encourage that but it is advisable to try it first with someone who has experienced it before.

Day	Cold shower	Breathing exercise	Retention time
1			
2			
3			
4			
5			
6			
7			
8			
9			
10			
11			
12			
13			
14			
15			
16			
17			
18			
19			
20			
21			
22			
23			
24			
25			
26			
27			
28			
29			
30			

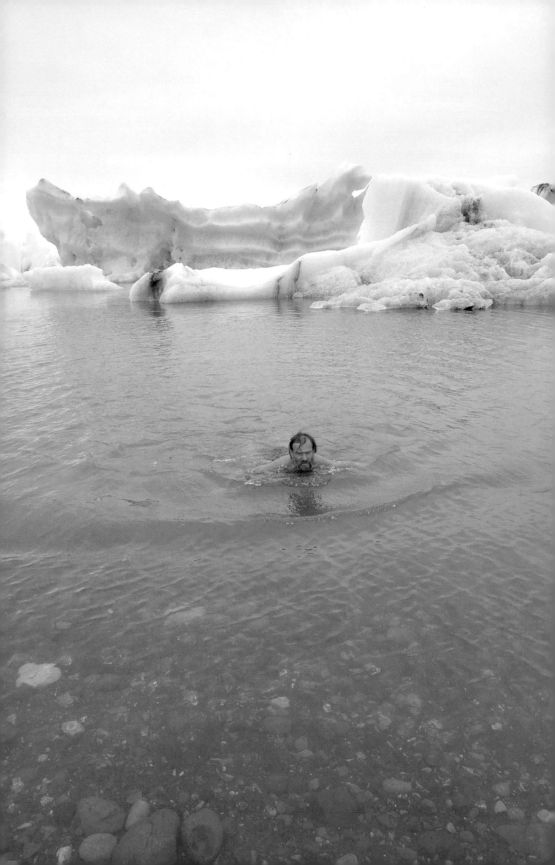

EPILOGUE

I t was December 17, 2014. I was walking along the Admiraal De Ruyterweg in Amsterdam in my swimming shorts and a t-shirt. It was 2°C (35.6°F) with a biting cold wind. Sleet whirled around in the air. I was walking from my house towards the Admiralengracht to take a dip. Ducks were swimming in the canal—they didn't mind the cold. I took off my t-shirt.

"Are you going swimming?" I heard a voice and looked around. A man wearing a winter hat, a thick raincoat, and a scarf pulled up high to cover his mouth looked at me in amazement.

"It's not really swimming," I answered. "I jump in the water and bob around for four or five minutes and then I get out again."

The man looked at me with his eyes popping out of his head. "That's really dangerous. Do you know how cold it is?"

I knew the exact temperature, because I'd measured it that same afternoon. "Four degrees," I replied.

The man is not reassured and doesn't want to read in the newspaper the next day that a man died of hypothermia in the Admiralengracht. So he waited. My explanation about Wim Hof, writing this book and doing cold training didn't completely convince him, but it aroused his curiosity. He asked me if he could film me. I told him that's fine, and lowered myself into the canal.

After a minute or two, the man was really enthusiastic. I bobbed around happily and explained all about blood vessels and the beneficial effects of the cold—all free of charge, and practically in our backyard. Excited, the man called his brother. He waved his arms around and told his brother that there really was someone swimming around in the canal and that he should come and take a look. It was very cold, it was snowing, and someone was bobbing around in the canal. As I climbed out of the canal and calmly put my t-shirt on, his brother walked up to us. I was soaking wet and with the ice-cold wind, I started to feel cold. I wanted to go home, but the brothers kept asking me one question after another. How was this possible? Why was I doing it? Should they do it? Who could benefit from it? Can everyone do it? I answered all their questions as best as I could. I wanted to satisfy their enthusiastic curiosity. The men walked off and called back that they would definitely read the book when it came out. At that time the book was still months in the future.

I went home and warmed up with a cup of tea. I understood how positive and gratifying Wim Hof's job of introducing curious people to the benefits of the cold really is.

A week later, I went for a swim in the Admiralengracht again. It was ten o'clock in the evening and dry, but still cold. It was dark and no one was on the street. I slid into the water, and after five minutes, I swam back to the side.

"What are you doing, sir?" I heard a deep voice ask from close by.

Two police officers looked at me suspiciously. They clearly wanted me to quickly account for my strange behavior. I explained that I was writing a book with Wim Hof, better known as the Iceman, and that of course I had to practice a little myself. The officers didn't seem very satisfied with this explanation, or with my swimming around in the canal. Didn't I know how dirty that water was? Of course, I'd had my doubts about it, but the canal water in Amsterdam has become a lot cleaner in recent years.

The police officers were still not very happy, and said that swimming in the canals was actually not allowed. Now I looked at them in surprise. You're not allowed to swim in the canals? I hadn't given it a second thought. They told me that there are 124 official swimming areas in the Province of North Holland, but that the Amsterdam canals were not among them.

"Oh," I answered. They let me go home with a warning, and a promise that I wouldn't do it again.

I went home, warmed myself up again with a cup of tea, and realized how difficult it is for Wim Hof to deal with skeptics and people who have a problem with all the special things he does.

I fervently hope that this book will help people rediscover the positive effects of the cold. And that it will build a bridge between Wim Hof and "normal" readers. Wim pushes the envelope and his enthusiasm comes from the depths of his soul. This sincerity can have a positive effect on some, but can also scare off other people. With this book, we want to show you that you don't have to go to Iceland to experience the benefits of cold. While writing it, I also sought out extremes—though not as extreme as Wim, of course—by swimming in the canal in the winter. But a cold shower will do just as well.

So, for now, warm—and cold—greetings,
— **Koen de Jong**
Nederhorst den Berg, February 2015

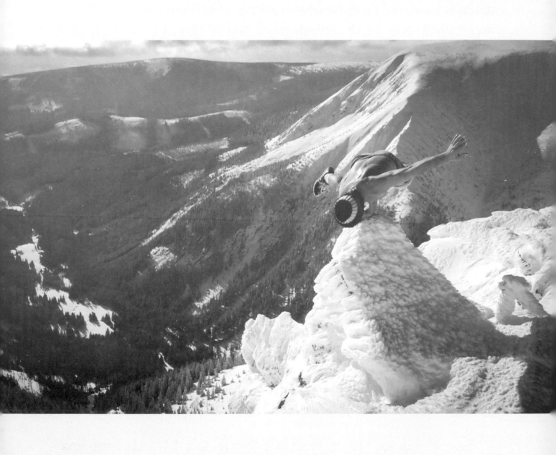

WORDS OF THANKS

WIM HOF

Who should I thank? Practically everyone. Thanks come from deep inside us—they are the forces that separates us from superficiality. It is a miracle how my message is spreading all around the world. Something so simple and yet, at the same time, so very, very strong. Believe in yourself and nature will thank you and yours, everyone, and our beautiful planet. I especially want to thank everyone who has supported me. With them, we will force back the coldness of disease and powerlessness even further.

KOEN DE JONG

In the first place, I would like to thank everyone who allowed me to interview them for this book. And I thank especially Mark Bos, Marianne Peper, Mathijs Storm, Richard de Leth and Jack Egberts for their candid and honest stories. Henk van den Bergh is not included as a profile in this book, but I would also like to thank him for his highly motivating enthusiasm.

Special thanks, too, to Professor Pierre Capel for his time and patience and his contribution to the chapter on the scientific underpinnings of the WHM. Our morning meetings were very elucidating and the evening we spent together with René Gude was special and informative.

I would also like to thank Stans van der Poel. She put me in touch with Pierre Capel. Without her, I never would have found out about him. I also thank her for her contribution to the chapter on breathing.

Enahm Hof, thanks for the coffee and the wonderful trip to Poland. Keep up the good work.

Lastly, I would like to thank the following for their close cooperation and contributions to this book: Bart Pronk, Robert Schraders (for helping me when I wrote off my car), Rob van Eupen, Bram Bakker, Dr. Geert Buijze, Linda Koeman, Maarten de Jong, Mark Zuurhout, Isabelle Hof (who had already described the method), and my blog teacher Kitty Kilian.

And the three of 241: Pauline Overeem, Palden Lama Overeem and Marin Koenszoon Overeem.

ABOUT THE AUTHORS

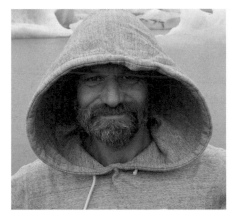

WIM HOF

Wim Hof is a Dutch daredevil who currently holds 20 world records relating to his ability to withstand extreme cold. As co-author of *Becoming the Iceman*, through his scientifically validated achievements and as the creator of the Wim Hof Method, he has inspired ten of thousands worldwide to reclaim their vitality through the practice of breath control and ice therapy.

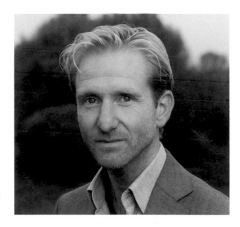

KOEN DE JONG

Koen de Jong lives in Amsterdam and has written six books about breathing and running. His book *The Marathon Revolution* is a bestseller in the Netherlands. He has run six marathons and is a practitioner of Vipassana meditation. Since meeting Wim Hof Koen enjoys winter swimming and his favorite book is *Momo* by Michael Ende.

Further Reading

In this book, we have tried to be as complete as possible. You can begin just by using the information and tips we have given you. Below is a list of websites and books where you can find out more.

Websites

WWW.INNERFIRE.NL

Wim and Enahm Hof's website has all the latest news on the scientific research into the WHM. You can also find Wim's program of lectures, workshops and organized trips.

WWW.WIMHOFMETHOD.COM

Here you will find an online course to take you through the WHM step-by-step in ten weeks. There are video clips and instructions on Wim Hof's breathing exercises and cold training. During the ten-week period, you can ask questions about your experiences.

WWW.COOLCHALLENGE.NL (CURRENTLY ONLY IN DUTCH)

On this site you can find the results of the research into the effects of cold showering conducted by the Academic Medical Centre in Amsterdam in January 2015. It also has regular blogs and background articles on the benefits of cold training.

WWW.SPORTRUSTEN.NL (CURRENTLY ONLY IN DUTCH)

On this site you can find information on breathing and breathing exercises at rest for relaxation. It also has a simple test to see how often you are breathing.

WWW.PUBMED.COM

This is an online library of scientific research into a wide range of medical topics, including the benefits of cold, breathing, and heart rate variability.

BOOKS

Healing without Freud or Prozac, David Servan-Schreiber (Rodale, 2011)

Verademing, Bram Bakker and Koen the Jong (Uitgeverij Lucht 2009) (in Dutch)

Yoga, Immortality and Freedom, Mircea Eliade (Bollingen-Princeton 1958)

De parasympaticus, in relatie met stress, geestelijke en lichamelijke ziekten, Pieter Langendijk and Agnes van Enkhuizen (Ankh Hermes 1989) (in Dutch)

A Life Worth Breathing, Max Strom (Skyhorse, 2010)

Teach Us To Sit Still, Tim Parks (Vintage Books, 2011)

GLOSSARY OF TERMS

Aerobic dissimilation: Aerobic dissimilation refers to the combustion of organic molecules—most often glucose, a much-used source of energy in organisms. During the aerobic dissimilation of glucose, glucose molecules are completely broken down into carbon dioxide and water molecules.

Aorta: The aorta is the main artery in the body. It starts in the left ventricle of the heart, and runs alongside the spinal cord to the abdomen. In an adult human, the aorta is 2-3 centimeters (0.8-1.2 inches) in diameter. While a person is at rest, around 5 liters (1.3 gallons) of blood flow through it per minute.

Ashram: An ashram is the Indian name for a living community and meeting place for members of a religious group. The word is often used in Hinduism to refer to a place of religious learning, frequently a monastery, or place of other religious significance. Mostly, an ashram will also be the home of a holy man. Ashrams were traditionally located far from areas of human habitation.

ATP: ATP stands for adenosine triphosphate, which plays a key role in the body as a source of chemical energy. The concentration of ATP in a cell ranges from 1 to 10 millimolar. A person weighing 70 kilograms (154 pounds) uses around 65 kilograms (143 pounds) of ATP a day while the quantity of ATP in the body at any given moment—free ATP—is only 50 grams (1.8 ounces). Cells therefore continuously produce ATP.

Autodidact: Someone who has taught him or herself through self-study and without supervision from a teacher or educational institution. The term is primarily used for self-teaching the equivalent of a substantial education, such as at university or a similarly high level.

Autoimmune disease: A disease in which the body attacks itself and is the cause of its own sickness. They occur when the immune system, designed to defend the body against intruders, produces antibodies to attack its own cells and tissues by mistake. We become sick because the body is trying to protect us from ourselves.

Autonomic nervous system: The autonomic nervous system regulates processes in the body such as temperature, heart rate, blood pressure, breathing, the dilation and contraction of the blood vessels, and the workings of the digestive system. The term autonomic suggests that we cannot influence these processes, but Wim Hof has conclusively shown that this is possible. The autonomic nervous system consists of two parts: the sympathetic and the parasympathetic systems.

Blood platelets: Blood platelets (thrombocytes) ensure that the blood coagulates. If a blood vessel is damaged, the platelets bind to the vessel wall and to each other, forming a scab that seals the leak. People with a deficit of blood platelets can suffer severe hemorrhaging.

Brown fat tissue: One of the two types of fat tissue found in mammals. Unlike white fat tissue, which primarily acts as energy storage, the main function of brown fat tissue is to generate body heat by burning fatty acids and glucose. Brown fat owes its name to the large quantity of mitochondria in its cells—many more than in the white fat tissue cells—which give it a brown color. Brown fat tissue only occurs in mammals.

Buteyko, Konstantin: Buteyko (Ukraine, 1923-2003) devised the method that bears his name. He determined that a carbon dioxide deficiency in the alveoli caused cramping of the blood vessels (hypertension) and of the bronchi (asthma). This led to the treatment known as the Buteyko method.

Capillaries: Capillaries are ultra-thin blood vessels.

Chromosomes: A chromosome is a DNA molecule and contains all of an individual's genetic information. Every cell in the body contains the same chromosomes. The genetic information is stored in the form of DNA strings. The pieces of DNA that contain this information are known as genes. Genes are always found in the same place in a chromosome in individuals of the same species.

Conditioning: Conditioning is a form of teaching, where linking two stimuli causes the response to one of the stimuli to change. It was first described by Russian researcher Ivan Pavlov. While studying the digestive processes of dogs, Pavlov discovered that they started salivating before he gave them food. He investigated this phenomenon further, to see whether he could teach the dogs to salivate unconsciously. He did this by ringing a bell five seconds before he fed the dogs. After doing this a few times, he observed that the dogs associated the bell with being fed. Soon, they started salivating when they heard the bell, without any food present.

Corpuscles, red and white: Red corpuscles (erythrocytes) are the most common form of corpuscles. They transport oxygen through the body with the aid of hemoglobin, a protein that is an excellent carrier of oxygen. Hemoglobin binds with oxygen easily, through iron. A shortage of hemoglobin and iron is known as anemia. The main function of white corpuscles (leukocytes) is to protect the body against everything foreign to it. In the event of a blood transfusion, the white corpuscles produce antibodies to combat the white corpuscles of the donor blood. In the best possible scenario, the patient suffers no ill effects from this process, but the antibodies can often cause a fever or worse side effects. To prevent this, the white corpuscles are filtered out of the donor blood as much as possible. This filtering process, known as leukocyte depletion, is applied during all blood transfusions.

Corticosteroids: These anti-inflammatory drugs are similar to a hormone produced by the body in the adrenal gland cortex. They are prescribed to combat various health problems and joint damage caused by rheumatism. Well-known corticosteroids are prednisone and prednisolone.

Cortisol: Known as the stress hormone, cortisol is released during all forms of stress, both physical and psychological. It is not the only stress hormone. Cortisol ensures that certain proteins in muscles are broken down, releasing amino acids from which glucose (energy) can be generated. This energy can be used to bring the body back into equilibrium. At the moment of stress, adrenaline and noradrenaline are released to make the body more alert and ready for "fight or flight". Cortisol ensures that this loss of energy can be replenished. Cortisol is produced in the adrenal gland cortex. The quantity produced follows a biological rhythm, meaning that it is not the same at every moment of the day. More is released when the body wakes up, making us feel hungry.

Creatine phosphate: Creatine phosphate (CP) is part of the body's anaerobic metabolism. It is a high-energy chemical that is stored in the muscle cells. CP is naturally produced in the body and is also found in foods like meat and fish. It ensures that the muscles contract when we start moving. During intense physical activity, CP releases energy quickly through a chemical reaction in which the phosphate is separated. The energy is used to further contract the muscles. Part of the creatine is then released into the blood and expelled from the body in the urine. The rest is absorbed by the muscles, via the liver, to provide more energy at a later stage. It is a self-regenerating system.

Cytokines: Molecules that play a role in the immune system and activate certain receptors. There are various kinds of cytokines which are released by different cells of the body. Some are produced constantly, while others are only released by cells activated during an immune response. The quantity of cytokines also varies, with some working only locally and others throughout the whole body.

Fast-5 diet: This "diet" was (re)discovered by former Air Force doctor Bert Herring. The regimen instructs you to only eat during a five-hour period each day, allowing your digestive system to rest during the remaining hours.

Glucose: Glucose is one of the human body's main sources of energy. Since it cannot be stored in the body, it is converted into glycogen, a polymer of glucose monomers stored in the muscles and the liver. Around 100 grams are stored in the average human body.

Hemoglobin: Hemoglobin is a protein in the blood of humans and many other animals. It binds with oxygen (oxyhemoglobin) to give blood its red color. Hemoglobin accounts for a third of the content of red corpuscles and is responsible for the transport of oxygen and carbon dioxide via the blood.

Heart rate variability: Heart rate variability refers to the variation in time between two successive heartbeats. Low HRV is a reliable indicator of stress.

Hypothalamus: The hypothalamus is part of the brain's limbic system. It controls the autonomic nervous system and plays a crucial role in organizing the actions that ensure the survival of the individual and the species, such as eating, fighting, fleeing and mating. It is also important in regulating the body's temperature.

Immune system: This is a defense mechanism designed to combat intruders and mutated cells in the body. The Latin term "immunis" means "exempt", and refers to protection from intruders. The body's immune system is actually an immune response involving multicellular organisms—a large number of cells and molecules work together to attack intruders. Besides protecting us against viruses, bacteria and parasites, the immune system also expels waste chemicals or cancerous and other sick cells from the body.

Lactate: Lactate is produced in muscles, the brain, and other tissues when there is too little oxygen present. Nutrients are absorbed in the body and burned in these organs to supply energy. Oxygen is necessary for good combustion. If sufficient oxygen is available, little or no lactate is produced. But if there is insufficient oxygen, lactate is produced during the combustion process instead of carbon dioxide and water. The lactate is then converted into carbon dioxide and water as soon as sufficient oxygen returns. If that takes too long, however, the lactate accumulates in the blood, disrupting the acid-alkali balance, causing the pH value to drop and leading to acidification.

Melatonin: Melatonin is a hormone produced in the pineal gland from serotonin then released into the blood and cerebrospinal fluid. The quantity released varies depending on the time of day. In many animals, it influences the sleep-wake and reproductive rhythms. In humans, the natural production of melatonin is directly linked to the certain retina receptors' exposure to light. Exposure to blue light (from sunlight or artificially from a television or a computer monitor) inhibits the production of melatonin. If the exposure to blue light decreases, the natural production of melatonin increases again. This is a signal for the body to reduce activity and prepare for sleep.

Microglia: Microglia are cells found in the macrophages of the central nervous system. They are small cells with a small core. Their cytoplasm contains a large number of lysosomes and other inclusions that are also found in other macrophages. Microglia occur in both the white and the grey matter of the central nervous system.

Mitochondria: Mitochondria are the powerhouses of the cell. As they supply cells with energy, there is a link between a cell's energy requirement and the number of mitochondria it contains.

Neocortex: The neocortex is the most recently evolved part of the brain. Relatively speaking, humans have a large neocortex compared to other mammals. It is home to our language center, our ability to think rationally, and our analytical capacity.

Oxygen saturation: Oxygen saturation indicates the percentage of hemoglobin bound to oxygen in the blood. This percentage should normally be 95% to 100%. Oxygen saturation refers only to the blood oxygen levels in the arteries. It does not indicate the replenishment of air in the lungs or the expulsion of carbon dioxide.

Parasympathetic system: This part of the nervous system is linked to relaxation, and is referred to as the body's "brake pedal". When it is active, the heart rate is low and breathing is calm. The digestive system is active and blood circulation is good.

Pineal gland: The pineal gland, or epiphysis cerebri, produces the hormone melatonin. This hormone influences various bodily functions. For example, we produce melatonin when there is insufficient daylight, which may also relate to our varying states of mind in different seasons. We need sufficient daylight (sunlight) to produce enough melatonin, which is released by the pineal gland if our sleep rhythm is correct.

Pituitary gland: This important organ just underneath the brain is the size of a pea—about 1 cm (0.4 inches) in diameter. It weighs no more than half a gram and is located in a cavity at the base of the skull. In a stressful situation, the pituitary gland releases a hormone called corticotropin which ensures that the adrenal glands produce cortisol. During this stress response, the pituitary gland is activated by the hypothalamus>. This interaction, known as the hypothalamic pituitary adrenal (HPA) axis, is a slow response to stress—it takes about 30 minutes before cortisol can be measured in the blood.

Plasma: Plasma consists of proteins, minerals, fats and hormones dissolved in water. It transports the corpuscles through the body and contains hundreds of different proteins—each with a different function. For example, the protein albumin absorbs water, ensuring that it stays in the blood vessels rather than leaching through to the tissues. Plasma also contains coagulating proteins which, together with blood platelets, play an important role in the coagulation process of blood.

Prednisone: prednisone is an anti-inflammatory drug.

PSA: The prostate-specific antigen is a protein normally present in the blood in small quantities. It is produced in the gland tissue of the prostate. It is not yet clear why PSA values vary, but it probably indicates activity in certain parts of the prostate tissue. We know that PSA values can increase with age without signifying irregularities of the prostate.

Receptors: Specific molecules can bind with these proteins in the cell membrane or the cell core. Receptors can receive signals from inside or outside the cell. When a signal molecule binds with a receptor, the receptor can initiate a cellular response. Both endogenous substances, such as neurotransmitters, hormones and cytokines, and exogenous ones like antigens and pheromones can stimulate such a cellular response.

Respiratory rate: This is the number of times that you breathe in a minute. Each breath begins as you start to breathe in and ends when you stop breathing out.

Sympathetic nervous system: This part of the nervous system is linked to action, and is known as the body's "accelerator". If this system is dominant, then we are in "fight-or-flight" mode. We breathe faster, our digestive system stops working momentarily, and our heart rate increases.

Telomeres: A telomere is a piece of DNA at the extreme end of a chromosome. It becomes shorter each time the cell divides. Telomeres protect DNA—after 50 or 60 times, a cell can no longer divide as the telomere is too short.

Transcription factors: A transcription factor is a protein that binds to the promoter of a gene. It controls the rate of transcription.

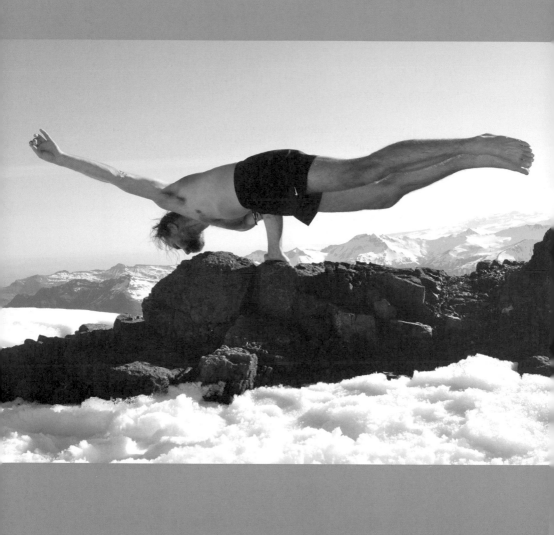

Consulted Literature and Research

LITERATURE

Dehue, Trudy, *De depressie-epidemie*, Atlas Contact 2010 (in Dutch).

Langendijk, Pieter and Van Enkhuizen, Agnes, *De parasympathicus, in relatie met stress, geestelijke en lichamelijke ziekten*, Ank Hermes 1989 (in Dutch).

Servan-Schreiber, David, *Healing without Freud or Prozac*, Rodale 2011.

Van der Poel, Stans, *Chronische vermoeidheid nooit meer*, Uitgeverij Lucht 2014 (in Dutch).

RESEARCH

Bleakly et al. "Onderzoek naar de effecten van koudwaterbaden op het herstel." www.ncbi.nlm.nih.gov/pubmed/20457737

David P. Fairlie, PhD. "Onderzoek naar verband tussen ontstekingen en overgewicht." www.fasebj.org/content/27/12/4757.abstract

Lobke Gierman "Inflammation: a link between metabolic syndrome and ostcoarthritis?" Dissertation, 2013.

Hopman et al. "Metabolisme van Hof tijdens blootstelling aan ijs stijgt met 300 procent." (2010) www.pubmed.com

Marken-Lichtenbeld et al. "Maar het blijkt dat bruin vetweefsel door kou kan worden geactiveerd." (2011) www.pubmed.com dioxide and water molecules.